T0325135

Delusions

Delusions

Understanding the Un-understandable

Peter McKenna
FIDMAG Hermanas Hospitalarias Research Foundation, Barcelona and the CIBERSAM research network, Spain

Figures drawn/redrawn
by Billie Wilson

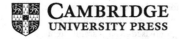

CAMBRIDGE
UNIVERSITY PRESS

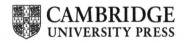

Shaftesbury Road, Cambridge CB2 8EA, United Kingdom

One Liberty Plaza, 20th Floor, New York, NY 10006, USA

477 Williamstown Road, Port Melbourne, VIC 3207, Australia

314–321, 3rd Floor, Plot 3, Splendor Forum, Jasola District Centre, New Delhi – 110025, India

103 Penang Road, #05–06/07, Visioncrest Commercial, Singapore 238467

Cambridge University Press is part of Cambridge University Press & Assessment,
a department of the University of Cambridge.

We share the University's mission to contribute to society through the pursuit of
education, learning and research at the highest international levels of excellence.

www.cambridge.org
Information on this title: www.cambridge.org/9781107075443

DOI: 10.1017/9781139871785

First published 2017

A catalogue record for this publication is available from the British Library

Library of Congress Cataloging-in-Publication data
Names: McKenna, Peter (Psychology) author.
Title: Delusions: understanding the un-understandable / Peter McKenna, FIDMAG Hermanas Hospitalarias
Research Foundation, Barcelona and the CIBERSAM research network, Spain; figures by Billie Wilson.
Description: Cambridge, United Kingdom; New York, NY: Cambridge University Press, 2017. |
Includes bibliographical references and index.
Identifiers: LCCN 2017008243 | ISBN 9781107075443 (hardback)
Subjects: LCSH: Delusions. | BISAC: MEDICAL / Mental Health.
Classification: LCC RC553.D35 M35 2017 | DDC 616.89–dc23
LC record available at https://lccn.loc.gov/2017008243

ISBN   978-1-107-07544-3   Hardback

....

Dedicated to the memory of Richard Marley, my commissioning editor at Cambridge University Press ... for encouraging me to write the book in the first place.

Contents

Preface

To a significant extent, this book came about as a result of a series of encounters with different people, the majority of which occurred by chance.

The first and the least random encounter was with my editor at Cambridge University Press Richard Marley. Sometime after a colleague, Tomasina Oh, and I had written a book that he had handled, he and I were talking casually about a possible next project. At some point in the conversation he said something along the lines of, 'What about a book on delusions?'.

A year or so later, having just moved to an academic job in Glasgow, and still labouring under the delusion that universities valued output in the form of books (which actually come a distant third after grants and papers in high-impact journals, at least in medical faculties), I sat down to write an outline for such a book. Then I sat down to do it again two or three more times. Each time it seemed flat; the more I wrote, the more I felt I was committing myself to a stodgy review of a large set of experimental psychological studies which had had less than electrifying findings.

What propelled the book forward during this period was a meeting with a psychiatrist colleague, Millia Begum. She asked for my comments on a review article she had nearly finished on an uncommon disorder, the olfactory reference syndrome. In Cambridge, I had previously been a regular attender at meetings that the distinguished historian of psychiatry, German Berrios, used to hold in his home, and from him I had learnt that the only way to really advance knowledge on uncommon disorders was to do a systematic review of all the reported cases in the world literature. It took us two years and Millia had to make several trips to Barcelona, where I had since moved to, but we finally managed to do this. Her enthusiasm (and our many arguments) rekindled an interest I had had thirty years ago in the distinction between delusions and overvalued ideas. She also introduced me to the knots DSM-IV was tying itself in over the classification of body dysmorphic disorder (not resolved in DSM-5). So if nothing else, this book owes a debt of gratitude to her.

Some time in 2012, it occurred to me that the best way to deal with the problems of a book on delusions was to try and write a draft of it and see how it looked. By then I had been working in Barcelona for four years and had met with the next person in the chain, Victor Vicens. He had the idea of doing an imaging study of delusional disorder, something I was sceptical about given that it is such an uncommon disorder. He also kept telling me that many such patients showed comorbidity with major affective disorder, something I was if anything even more sceptical about. I was half-right about the former – it took us several years to find and scan 22 patients with delusional disorder – and completely wrong about the latter. The relationship with affective disorder, which is almost one that dare not speak its name (it is referred without any explanation in DSM-III-R through DSM-5 and in ICD-10), made me think that someone ought to at least try and say something about the existence and implications of the association.

This brings me to the last encounter, which really was completely by chance. Wolfram Hinzen, a philosopher and linguist, came to work in Barcelona on an international fellowship. I will never forget our first meeting, where he explained to me how he thought formal thought disorder was definitely due to a problem with grammar. Since Tomasina Oh and I had argued strongly in our previous Cambridge University Press book that syntax was not affected in patients with the symptom, this was not exactly what I wanted to hear. Fortunately, it turned out that what he meant by grammar was something deeper and more wide ranging than syntax, so honour was satisfied. Together with another colleague, Joana Rosselló, we went on to have an extended series of discussions about delusions in the tapas bars (and sometimes just the bars) of Barcelona. It is fair to say that without Wolfram's input, what this book says on dopamine and the salience theory would have been considerably less thought through than it is, and I probably wouldn't have been able to say anything much at all about several issues raised in the final chapter.

Other people who deserve thanks are Tony David for discussions about delusions and pointing me to Gray's response to Kapur's article on aberrant salience, and more importantly for being one of the editors of the journal *Cognitive Neuropsychiatry*, without which the literature on delusions would be considerably poorer. While I was in Glasgow I also met Sammy Jauhar, who I went on to collaborate with and who has been a continual source of support, not to mention getting hold of many papers and book chapters that I couldn't access. Benedikt Amann was kind enough to translate Wernicke's original writing on overvalued ideas. Last but not least, three years or so ago, I started spending some of my time in Yorkshire, coincidentally about 20 minutes' drive from the British Library Document Store in Boston Spa. This has a reading room with very friendly staff, who repeatedly went out of their way to help me get the papers that not even Sammy Jauhar could access. *Israel Annals of Psychiatry and Allied Disciplines* in the 1960s – no problem!

So, eight years after I first started thinking about it, I finally sent Richard Marley an outline of a book on delusions. He was gracious enough to approve it. Sadly, he did not live to see the final product, as he died prematurely in 2016.

The book does not work towards a theory of delusions. Instead I have tried to tell a story which has various themes that overlap without interlocking particularly. Nor should the fact that the penultimate chapter is on the salience theory be taken to imply that I think this is more important than other approaches to delusions (though I admit to having a certain weakness for it). In the end, writing the book turned out to be a more interesting exercise than I anticipated. At any rate, I hope the result isn't too stodgy.

What Is a Delusion?

Delusions have always presented a particular challenge for psychiatry. It is not just that they are such an arresting phenomenon – patients with schizophrenia, the main but by no means the only disorder where they are seen, routinely make claims that are completely impossible but are narrated in a completely matter-of-fact way – it is also because they are central to the concepts of sanity and insanity in a way that other symptoms of mental illness are not. As the psychiatrist and philosopher Jaspers (1959) put it in a quote that has been repeated so many times it is in danger of becoming a cliché: 'Since time immemorial, delusion has been taken as the basic characteristic of madness. To be mad was to be deluded.'

The first step in understanding any phenomenon is to define it. However, in the case of delusions, this has not proved easy to do. Of course, like other psychiatric symptoms they have a textbook definition: they are false beliefs which are fixed, incorrigible and out of keeping with the individual's social and cultural background. Unfortunately, as Jaspers and a steady stream of later authors have pointed out, criteria of fixity and incorrigibility are not very helpful when it seems to be a universal human characteristic to hold on stubbornly to beliefs that are often self-evidently wrong. The part of the definition about the belief being out of keeping with the individual's social and cultural background might also be considered slightly suspect, given that it seems to leave a lot to the subjective judgement of the clinician. This and several other definitional problems were pithily summed up by David (1999):

> [D]espite the facade created by psychiatric textbooks, there is no acceptable (rather than accepted) definition of a delusion. Most attempted definitions begin with 'false belief', and this is swiftly amended to an unfounded belief to counter the circumstance where a person's belief turns out to be true. Then caveats accumulate concerning the person's culture and whether the beliefs are shared. Religious beliefs begin to cause problems here and religious delusions begin to create major conflicts. The beleaguered psychopathologist then falls back on the 'quality' of the belief – the strength of the conviction in the face of contradictory evidence, the 'incorrigibility', the personal commitment, etc. Here, the irrationality seen in 'normal' reasoning undermines the specificity of these characteristics for delusions as does the variable conviction and fluctuating insight seen in patients with chronic psychoses who everyone agrees are deluded. Finally we have the add-ons: the distress caused by the belief, its preoccupying quality, and its maladaptiveness generally, again, sometimes equally applicable to other beliefs held by non-psychotic fanatics of one sort or another. In the end we are left with a shambles.

Even if these problems are capable of resolution, simply defining delusions fails to do something at least as important, that of communicating what the experience of being deluded is like. This problem is easier to put right, since there is a reasonably substantial descriptive literature on the symptom. In fact, one needs to look no further than the accounts of Kraepelin (1913a,b) and Bleuler (1911; 1924) to get a vivid and very detailed account of what deluded patients actually say. Later, Jaspers (1959) contributed additional important descriptions of his own. Beyond this, it is slightly surprising to realize that there is really one major contemporary source of original material. This had its origins in a drive that took place in the 1960s and 1970s to make the notoriously unreliable assessment of psychiatric symptoms more objective, which resulted in the development of a series of structured interviews for schizophrenia and other disorders. One of these stood out in terms of the broadness of its reach and sophistication of its psychopathological description. This was the Present State Examination (PSE) of Wing and co-workers (1974) and it had a particularly rich and detailed section on delusions.

Of course, it was never just a matter of description. Both Kraepelin and Bleuler had something to say about how and why delusions might arise. Jaspers became famous for trying to capture the essential nature of abnormal subjective experiences using a method called phenomenology. The conclusions he came to about delusions have had a lasting impact, although, as will be seen, they led to a disagreement with another phenomenologically minded author of the day, Schneider (1949). As Wing et al. (1974) refined their classification of delusions over nine editions of the PSE (there is now also a tenth), they also sometimes found themselves providing their own pragmatic solutions to a number of problems left over from the classical era.

This chapter describes the diverse clinical features of delusions, focusing on the contributions of the aforementioned authors. Their various attempts to go further and capture something of the essential nature of delusions, as well as the disputes that sometimes arose between them, provide a kind of parallel discourse that hopefully also allows something to be said about delusions beyond just defining them. Tricky questions about what is and is not a delusion are sidestepped for the time being by limiting the discussion to beliefs that everyone would agree are obviously delusional.

Describing Delusions: Kraepelin and Bleuler

Despite being written more than a century ago in another language, Kraepelin's descriptions of psychotic symptoms have an immediacy that has never been equalled. In the seventh edition of his textbook of psychiatry (Kraepelin, 1907), he began with what would now be regarded as a rather undifferentiated conception of *persecutory delusions*: patients would feel they were being watched, they would observe peculiar acts in public places that referred to them, children on the street would jeer and laugh at them wherever they went, all of which led them to believe that people were conspiring against them. *Hypochondriacal or somatic delusions* were another prominent type. Patients would express beliefs that their intestines were shrinking or that their organs had been removed, often bound up with the imagined persecution. *Expansive or grandiose delusions* were also seen and could be as varied as the ideas of persecution and bodily change. Patients would say that they had been awarded a prize for bravery, that they ruled the country, or that they were talented poets or the greatest inventor ever born; or alternatively that they had God-like attributes, had been transformed into Christ, would ascend to heaven and so on. What Kraepelin called ideas of spirit-possession often went hand in hand with these other kinds of delusions. Here the persecutor or persecutors would enter and take control of the body, causing the patient's bones to crack, his testicles to fall or his or her throat to dry up.

Kraepelin's multi-volume, eighth edition of his textbook (Kraepelin, 1913a,b) contained similar but more detailed descriptions. Where this later account really came into its own with respect to delusions, however, was in his account of paraphrenia and paranoia. Paraphrenia was the term he gave to a group of disorders closely related to schizophrenia, which were characterized by florid delusions and hallucinations but few if any other symptoms. His description of one of the subtypes of paraphrenia, paraphrenia systematica, is notable for how delusions, especially persecutory delusions, grew out of the experience of *referentiality*. At first:

> The patient notices that he is the object of general attention. On his appearance the neighbours put their heads together, turn round to look at him, watch him. On the street he is stared at; strange people follow him, look at one another, make signs to one another; policemen are standing about everywhere. In the restaurants to which he goes, his coming is already announced; in the newspapers there are allusions to him; the sermon is aimed at him; there must be something behind it all.

At the same time, people's motives would seem to be anything but friendly:

> [E]verything is done to spite him; people work systematically against him. The servants are incited against him, cannot endure him any longer; the children have no longer any respect for him; people are trying to remove him from his situation, to prevent him from marrying, to undermine his existence, to drive him into the night of insanity. Female patients perceive that people are trying to dishonour them, to seduce them, to bring them to shame.

Slowly, sometimes over the course of years, the reason for the persecution would become more and more tangible:

> Obviously there exists a regular conspiracy that carries on the persecution; sometimes it is the social democrats, the 'red guard', sometimes the Freemasons, sometimes the Jesuits, the Catholics, the spiritualists, the German Emperor, the 'central union', the members of the club, the neighbours, the relatives, the wife, but especially former mistresses, who cause all the mischief.

There was no such logical progression in what Kraepelin termed paraphrenia phantastica. As its name suggests, this was characterized by the spontaneous appearance of *fantastic delusions*. These could be persecutory, grandiose or hypochondriacal in nature, but their main feature was their wholly absurd content and the way in which they were produced in a seemingly inexhaustible supply. Patients would express the beliefs that there were multiple other people inside them or that they owned properties on other planets. One patient believed that a whole car had entered his body, with the steering wheel sticking out of his ears. Another talked about an international conspiracy that existed for getting rid of people by means of lifts in hotels, which took them down into subterranean vaults, where a sausage machine was waiting for them.

In a small group of cases ('paraphrenia confabulans'), the patients produced, in addition to other delusions and sometimes hallucinations, detailed accounts of fictitious events, something Kraepelin called pseudo-memories but are now referred as *delusional memories* and *delusional confabulations*. One patient related how, as a child, he had been taken to the Royal Palace where he was shown the room where he was born and later met one of the King's daughters who promised to marry him. Another patient went to the police and reported that he had dug up a human arm (which resulted in a police investigation). Sometimes the fictitious events would be repeated almost word for word on different occasions, but in other cases the tale would be continually embroidered. For example, the patient who stated he had dug up an arm later went on to recount how his mother and other individuals in the village had disappeared, and that a woman in the neighbourhood had threatened him with a gun and said that it would be his turn next.

Delusions were not just a feature of schizophrenia and paraphrenia. They also occurred in the states that Kraepelin (1913a, b) brought together as manic-depressive insanity (a term which would now cover bipolar disorder and unipolar major depression). In the mildest form of mania, hypomania, it was more a case of exaggerations and distortions than delusions: patients boasted about their aristocratic acquaintances and prospects of marriage, gave themselves non-existent titles, and had visiting cards printed with a crown on them. These ideas gave way to fully fledged delusions in more severely affected cases – the patients were geniuses, were of noble or royal descent, possessed great riches, were saints, Jesus or God – although the beliefs could still sometimes be fleeting or expressed in half-joking way.

In depression, the same range of abnormal beliefs was seen in mirror image, from unfounded gloomy and self-depreciatory thoughts in what he called 'melancholia simplex', through to undoubted delusions playing on the same themes. In these latter cases, patients would say things like they were the most wicked person, an abomination, or had committed fraud and would be imprisoned for 10 years. Others believed they were incurably ill with cancer or syphilis and/or they were making people around them ill. A heartrending example of what are now referred to as *depressive delusions* is given in Box 1.1.

Box 1.1 Extract from a Letter by a Female Patient with Depressive Delusions to Her Sister (Kraepelin, 1913b)

I wish to inform you that I have received the cake. Many thanks, but I am not worthy. You sent it on the anniversary of my child's death, for I am not worthy of my birthday; I must weep myself to death; I cannot live and I cannot die, because I have failed so much, I shall bring my husband and children to hell. We are all lost; we won't see each other any more; I shall go to the convict prison and my two girls as well, if they do not make away with themselves, because they were borne in my body. If I had only remained single! I shall bring all my children into damnation, five children! Not far enough cut in my throat, nothing but unworthy confessions and communion; I have fallen and it never in my life occurred to me; I am to blame that my husband died and many others. God caused the fire in our village on my account; I shall bring many people into the institution. My good, honest John was so pious and has to take his life; he got nineteen marks on Low Sunday, and at the age of nineteen his life came to an end. My two girls are there, no father, no mother, no brother, and no one will take them because of their wicked mother. God puts everything into my mind; I can write to you a whole sheet full of nothing but significance; you have not seen it, what signs it has made. I have heard that we need nothing more, we are lost.

Note: 'Not far enough cut in my throat' referred to a suicide attempt the patient had made. John, her husband, was in fact alive.

Kraepelin was not quite finished with delusions yet. He argued that a small number of patients showed insidiously developing delusions in the absence of any other psychotic (or mood) symptoms and with little if any change in other areas of thinking. In this disorder, paranoia, the beliefs often, though not always, took a persecutory form and in many cases they followed a long period of suspiciousness and referentiality. The central delusion itself was also different from delusions in other disorders, in that it did not show gross internal contradictions and, despite its usual extreme unlikeliness, did 'not usually contain any apparent absolute impossibilities'. This idea survives to the present day as the concept of *non-bizarre delusions*.

Bleuler, Kraepelin's contemporary and the other towering psychiatric figure of the day, generally had less to say about delusions. In his book on schizophrenia (Bleuler, 1911), he described persecutory delusions as being particularly common, and emphasized the wide variety of organizations that were alleged to be involved, including the patients' fellow-employees, the Freemasons, the Jesuits, mind-readers and spiritualists, among others. In his experience, grandiose delusions were also common and usually occurred alongside persecutory delusions. He also noted that depressive delusions could be seen which were very similar to those described by Kraepelin in delusional forms of melancholia; sometimes they seemed to be related to the patient's current mood state, but this was by no means always the case.

There was no shortage of fantastic delusions in Bleuler's (1911) account. Patients could be animals, a frog, a dog, a shark, or even an inanimate object. Women gave birth to 150 children every night. A patient had human beings in her fingers who wanted to kill her and drink her blood. Hypochondriacal delusions, often with a bizarre or fantastic quality, were also common: patients would say things like there was a growth in their heads, their bones had turned to liquid, or that their bone marrow was running out in their sperm. He also drew attention to the occurrence of *sexual delusions*, as in male patients who felt they were female, and vice-versa.

Bleuler additionally highlighted a phenomenon, ideas of influence, that had only been noted in passing by Kraepelin:

> [T]hese hostile forces observe and note his every action and thought by means of 'mountain-mirrors', or by electrical instruments and influence him by means of mysterious apparatus and magic. They make the voices; they cause him every conceivable, unbearable sensation. They cause him to go stiff, deprive him of his thoughts or make him think certain thoughts … The bodily 'influencing' constitutes an especially unbearable torture for these patients. The physician stabs their eyes with a 'knife voice'. They are dissected, beaten, electrocuted; their brain is sawn in pieces, their muscles are stiffened. A constantly operating machine has been installed in their heads.

This class of delusions would go on to become a focus of much subsequent interest as one of the so-called first-rank symptoms of schizophrenia, *passivity* or *delusions of control*.

Like Kraepelin, Bleuler (1911; 1924) considered that delusions of reference could be an important starting point for the development of persecutory delusions. Patients with grandiose delusions had also often had vague and undefined great hopes and ambitions at the start of their illnesses, which then later assumed a more definite form. However, he did not feel that this mode of development could be established as a general principle. In some cases, the sudden appearance of sharply formulated ideas was the first symptom of the illness; in others, delusions appeared in consciousness all at once, as it were as finished products.

The Phenomenology of Delusions: Jaspers versus Schneider

Memorable though they were, Kraepelin's and Bleuler's descriptions of delusions were just that – descriptions. Neither author spent much time deliberating over the nature or limits of the phenomenon, or on features such as fixity and incorrigibility. It was Jaspers who more than anyone else shouldered this responsibility. He was the first and, it is probably fair to say, the only author to seriously grapple with the definition of delusion. He also formulated a theory of delusions whose influence rightly or wrongly is still felt today. Along the way he also contributed some fine descriptions of the symptom, especially with respect to referentiality.

Jaspers' thinking about delusions appeared in successive editions of his book *General Psychopathology*, the last of which was published in 1959. This version is long and mostly very dense (the only way the present author has ever been able to approach it is to look up topics in the index and read the relevant pages). Fortunately, his views on delusions have been lucidly summarized and explained by Walker (1991) in an article with the title 'Delusions: what did Jaspers really say?', and this will be drawn on repeatedly in what follows.

Jaspers started by exposing the deficiencies in the standard definition of delusions. He noted that the term tended to be applied to false judgements which showed the following external characteristics: (1) they are held with extraordinary conviction, an incomparable subjective certainty; (2) there is an imperviousness to other experiences and to compelling counter-argument; and (3) their content is impossible. He dismissed the first two features out of hand. Intensity of conviction neither distinguished delusions from normal strongly held scientific, political or ethical convictions, nor from the overvalued idea (a symptom that is discussed in detail in the next chapter). Nor was incorrigibility a good criterion, since normal wrong beliefs are also notoriously difficult to correct and are often clung on to tenaciously. This point was nicely made by Walker (1991):

> Imagine John Major and Neil Kinnock [the Prime Minister and leader of the opposition at the time] in full flow at the dispatch box of the House of Commons. Both hold views with an 'extraordinary conviction' and 'an incomparable subjective certainty'. Both show a very definite 'imperviousness to other experiences and to compelling counter-argument'. For each, the judgements of the other are 'false' and 'their content impossible'. Obviously, neither is deluded.

Jaspers also made the point that beliefs which otherwise showed all the characteristics of delusions were not necessarily held with full conviction. Patients' attitudes to their beliefs could range from a mere play with possibilities, through a 'double reality' where the real and the delusional existed side by side, to full conviction ('unequivocal attitudes in which the delusional content reigns as the sole and absolute reality').

Next, Jaspers went on to explore the nature of delusions. He did this using phenomenology, his own partly clinical, partly philosophical method for grasping the nature of psychotic and other psychiatric symptoms. The important features of the approach are summarized in Box 1.2, but ultimately it boiled down to abstracting the essential features of a particular abnormal subjective experience from the very varied descriptions that patients gave, while at the same time taking care not to impose unwarranted theoretical interpretations on the results of the exercise.

Box 1.2 Jaspers on Phenomenology (Jaspers, 1912, reproduced with permission from the British Journal of Psychiatry)

We must begin with a clear representation of what is actually going on in the patient, what he is really experiencing, how things arise in his consciousness, what are his own feelings, and so forth; and at this stage we must put aside altogether such considerations as the relationships between experiences, or their summation as a whole, and more especially we must avoid trying to supply any basic constructs or frames of reference. We should picture only what is really present in the patient's consciousness; anything that has not really presented itself to his consciousness is outside our consideration. We must set aside all outmoded theories, psychological constructs or materialist mythologies of cerebral processes; we must turn our attention only to that which we can understand as having real existence, and which we can differentiate and describe. This, as experience has shown, is in itself a very difficult task ...

The methods by which we carry out a phenomenological analysis and determine what patients really experience are of three kinds: (1) one immerses oneself, so to speak, in their gestures, behaviour, expressive movements; (2) exploration, by direct questioning of the patients and by means of accounts which they themselves, under our guidance, give of their own experiences; (3) written self-descriptions – seldom really good, but then all the more valuable; they can, in fact, be made use of even if one has not known the writer personally ...

So before real inquiry can begin it is necessary to identify the specific psychic phenomena which are to be its subject, and form a clear picture of the resemblances and differences between them and other phenomena with which they must not be confused. This preliminary work of representing, defining, and classifying psychic phenomena, pursued as an independent activity, constitutes phenomenology. The difficult and comprehensive nature of this preliminary work makes it inevitable that it should become for the time being an end in itself.

Psychopathological phenomena seem to call for just such an approach, one which will isolate, will make abstractions from related observations, will present as realities only the data themselves without attempting to understand how they have arisen; an approach which only wants to see, not to explain.

On phenomenological grounds, what Jaspers felt set delusions apart from other beliefs was a single, fundamental property: they were un-understandable. What he meant by un-understandability, however, turned out to be quite complicated. In one sense it simply meant that delusions – true delusions or delusions proper, as opposed to overvalued and other 'delusion-like' ideas – were psychologically irreducible; they did not emerge comprehensibly from anything else in the patient's current or past mental life, either normal ('shattering, mortifying, guilt-provoking or other such experiences') or pathological ('false-perception or from the experience of derealization in states of altered consciousness etc.'). As Walker (1991) later put it, Jaspers felt that delusions were not understandable in the sense of the normal empathic access that one has to another person's subjective experience using the analogy of one's own experience.

Un-understandability also included a dimension of being unmediated. As Walker (1991) explained, cutting through Jaspers' whole concept of phenomenology was the distinction between unmediated or immediate experiences and those that are the product of reflection. Unmediated experiences are elementary or irreducible, and are characterized by an immediate certainty of reality. In contrast, mediated experiences are judgements about the reality of these experiences which involve processes of thinking and working through. For Jaspers, delusions were not a product of reflection, and in a way they could even be considered to be an experience, although not in the perceptual sense of the term. This sense of un-understandable lay behind his use of phrases like 'the primary delusional experience', and delusion as something that 'comes before thought, although it becomes clear to itself only in thought'.

Could the nature of delusions be defined further? Jaspers thought that it could, although in doing so he went some way beyond the strict rules he himself had laid down for phenomenology. He proposed that delusions ultimately reflected a change in the way in which meaning is attached to events. The experience of events was, he argued, not just a mechanical perceptual process, there was always an accompanying sense of meaning: a house is seen as something that people inhabit, a knife as a tool for cutting and so on. In the case of delusions, perception itself remained normal, but the process of seeing of meaning underwent a radical transformation, so that it became immediate and intrusive. This altered sense of meaning was clearly evident in a symptom Jaspers described in the early stages of psychotic disorders, where the patient has an indefinable sensation that the world is changing or something suspicious is afoot, *delusional mood*:

> The environment is somehow different – not to a gross degree – perception is unaltered in itself but there is some change which envelops everything with a subtle, pervasive and strangely uncertain light. A living-room which formerly was felt as neutral or friendly now becomes dominated by some indefinable atmosphere. Something seems in the air which the patient cannot account for, a distrustful, uncomfortable, uncanny tension invades him.

Individual objects and events also started to signify something, although still nothing definite; they were simply eerie, horrifying, peculiar, or alternatively remarkable, mystifying or transcendental:

> A patient noticed the waiter in the coffee-house; he skipped past him so quickly and uncannily. He noticed odd behaviour in an acquaintance which made him feel strange; everything in the street was so different, something was bound to be happening. A passer-by gave such a penetrating glance, he could be a detective. Then there was a dog who seemed hypnotised, a kind of mechanical dog made of rubber. There were such a lot of people walking about, something must surely be starting up against the patient. All the umbrellas were rattling as if some apparatus was hidden inside them.

In what Jaspers implied was the next stage in this process, the patient arrived at defining these events as more clearly having some obvious relationship to him or her, or in other words as delusions of reference:

> Gestures, ambiguous words provide 'tacit intimations'. All sorts of things are being conveyed to the patient. People imply quite different things in such harmless remarks as 'the carnations are lovely' or 'the blouse fits all right' and understand these meanings very well among themselves. People look at the patient as if they had something special to say to him. – 'It was as if everything was being done to spite me; everything that happened in Mannheim happened in order to take it out of me.' People in the street are obviously discussing the patient. Odd words picked up in passing refer to him. In the papers, books, everywhere there are things which are specially meant for the patient, concern his own personal life and carry warnings or insults.

What Jaspers then went on to propose involved a conceptual leap: all other types of delusions were also characterized by the same changed awareness of meaning. In support of this view, he gave the example of a girl who was reading about Lazarus being woken from the dead in the Bible and immediately felt herself to be the Virgin Mary. She vividly experienced the events she had just read about as if they were her own experience, although this vividness did not have sensory qualities. However, while the belief that Jaspers described in this example was certainly sudden and intrusive, how it specifically involved a changed awareness of meaning was not made clear. The only further clarification Jaspers gave concerned another patient who suddenly had the notion that a fire had broken out in a faraway town. 'This', he argued 'surely happens only through the meaning he draws from inner visions that crowd in on him with the character of reality'. Walker (1991) was not overly impressed by this argument, describing it as lame.

Someone else who was not impressed was Schneider, the psychiatrist who delineated the first rank symptoms of schizophrenia. He (Schneider, 1949) distinguished between two types of delusion: on the one hand there were delusional perceptions (somewhat similar to delusions of reference, though they appeared suddenly and had a highly specific content), where abnormal significance became attached to a real event without any cause that was understandable in rational or emotional terms. On the other hand were what he referred to as delusional ideas and intuitions, which covered virtually all other types of delusions, including grandiose, religious and persecutory convictions and at least some beliefs about ill-health. He did not see how the concept of abnormal meaning could be extended to cover these latter delusions. In his slightly overcomplicated way of describing it:

> Delusional intuition does not consist in attributing unfounded significance to an actual percept: it is purely ideational ... If it comes into someone's head that he is Christ, that is a single process involving both the person and the intuition. There is no second part, extending from the perceived object (which includes normal comprehension and understandable interpretation) to the abnormal significance attached to it which goes with a delusional perception.

Nor did Schneider feel it was credible to argue that this latter class of delusion had a component of significance by virtue of the fact that the beliefs were often of momentous importance to the patient. This was to use the word significance in a very different sense from that of abnormal meaning being attached to a perceived event.

Delusions Today: Wing, Cooper and Sartorius

How has psychiatric thinking about delusions changed in the half-century or so since Jaspers and Schneider crossed swords over the role of meaning? On the face of it, not much. Textbooks and review articles continue to rehearse the standard definition that they are fixed, incorrigible beliefs which are out of keeping with the individual's culture and background. Two British authors, Sims (1988; 1995) and Cutting (1985), who wrote books on psychopathology with chapters on delusions, also did not stray far from the fold in this respect (and were duly chastised by Walker (1991) for this). But nowhere was the steadfast adherence to dogma more apparent than in the landmark *American Diagnostic and Clinical Manual of Mental Disorders, Third Edition*, (DSM-III). Its terse and superficial definition of delusions in the glossary gave the distinct impression that deep thinking about phenomenological issues was not welcome.

DSM-III itself was a response to a series of scandals about the loose way in which schizophrenia was being diagnosed, particularly in America. This led to the adoption of a criterion-based approach to diagnosis, something that is now routinely employed all over the world. According to this, psychiatric disorders are defined by the presence of a certain number of symptoms in certain combinations, together with the absence of other symptoms. Schizophrenia, for example, is diagnosed on the basis of the patient showing multiple delusions, or both delusions and hallucinations, or having pathognomonic symptoms (i.e. Schneiderian first rank symptoms), with the additional requirements that there are insufficient symptoms to diagnose a full affective disorder, and there is no evidence of organic brain disease.

Another response to the problem was the development of a series of so-called structured psychiatric interviews designed to elicit psychiatric symptoms in an unequivocal way.

The idea was that by asking patients a comprehensive set of precisely formulated questions, diagnostic practice in psychiatry could be placed on an equal footing with that in the rest of medicine. Most of these structured interviews were rather turgid affairs, plodding through a long series of questions covering in turn the symptoms of schizophrenia, mania, major depression and in some cases other disorders as well. One, however, was different; this was the Present State Examination (PSE) developed by Wing and his co-workers Cooper and Sartorius over more than ten years to emerge in its final form as its ninth edition in 1974 (Wing et al., 1974) (a tenth edition has since been released which is similar but covers a broader range of disorders). For a start, it was an order of magnitude more detailed than other structured interviews – rather than simply eliciting the symptoms necessary to make a diagnosis, its aim was to give a detailed picture of the patient's current symptomatology (or in its 'lifetime' form, the symptoms experienced over a period of months or years). Its section on delusions was particularly rich, including some forms of the symptom that would probably be unfamiliar to many clinicians. There was also a glossary of symptoms in the accompanying manual which, in sharp contrast to that provided at the end of DSM-III and its successors, provided useful practical information on every symptom rated. This additionally offered solutions to a number of phenomenological debates and uncertainties which, while typically pragmatic, often betrayed a sophisticated knowledge of the currents of historical thought.

Wing et al.'s (1974) classification of delusions in the ninth edition of the PSE is summarized in Box 1.3. It can be seen that those where neutral events have significance for the patient are multiply represented, as delusional mood and delusions of reference, misinterpretation and misidentification (this use of misidentification is different from that used to refer to the Capgras and related syndromes discussed in Chapter 7). A special case of this type of delusion is what the PSE calls primary delusions. This refers to an experience where a patient suddenly becomes convinced that a particular set of events has a special but also highly specific meaning. The example Wing et al. (1974) gave was of a patient undergoing a liver biopsy who, as the needle was being inserted, felt that he had been chosen by God. This symptom is more commonly known as *delusional perception*, following the views expressed by Schneider (1949) described in the previous section.

Box 1.3 The PSE Classification of Delusions (Wing, Cooper and Sartorius, 1974)

Delusions of Control

The subject's will is replaced by that of some external agency. He feels under the control of some force or power other than himself, as though he is a robot or a zombie or possessed. It makes his movements for him without him willing it, or uses his voice or his handwriting, or replaces his personality.

Delusional Mood

The subject feels that his familiar environment has changed in a way which puzzles him and which he may not be able to describe clearly. Everything feels odd, strange and uncanny, something suspicious is afoot, events are charged with new meaning. The state typically precedes the development of full delusions: the patient may fluctuate between acceptance and rejection of various delusional explanations, or the experience may suddenly crystallize into a clear, fully formed delusional idea.

Delusions of Reference

People drop hints about what the subject says, or says things with a double meaning, or do things in a special way so as to convey a special meaning. The whole neighbourhood may seem to be gossiping about him, far beyond the bounds of possibility, or he may see references to himself on the television or in newspapers. He may seem to be followed, his movements observed, and that what he says tape-recorded. There are people about who are not what they seem to be.

Delusions of Misinterpretation and Misidentification

This is an extension of the delusion of reference so that situations appear to be created which have a special meaning. Things seem to be specially arranged to test the patient out, objects are arranged so that they have a special significance for him, street signs or advertisements on buses or patterns of colour seem to have been put there in order to give him a message. Whole armies of people may seem to be employed simply in order to discover what he is doing, or to convey some message to him.

Delusions of Persecution

Someone is deliberately trying to harm him, e.g. poison him or kill him. The symptom may take many forms, from the direct belief that people are hunting him down, to complex and bizarre plots with every kind of science fiction.

Delusions of Assistance

The subject believes that someone, or some organization, or some force or power, is trying to help him. The beliefs may be simple (people make signs to the subject in order to persuade him to be a better person, because they want to help him) or complicated (angels organize everything so that the subject's life is directed in the most advantageous way).

Delusions of Grandiose Abilities

The subject believes he has special abilities or powers, e.g. he is much cleverer than anyone else, has invented machines, composed music or solved mathematical problems, etc., beyond most people's comprehension, or there is a special purpose or mission to his life.

Delusions of Grandiose Identity

The subject believes he is famous, rich, titled or related to prominent people.

Religious Delusions

The subject believes he is specially close to Christ or God, is a saint, has special spiritual powers, etc.

Delusional Explanations in Terms of Paranormal Phenomena

The subject is influenced by hypnotism, telepathy or the occult.

Delusional Explanations in Terms of Physical Forces

Electricity, X-rays, radio-waves or similar are affecting the subject.

Delusions of Alien Forces Penetrating or Controlling Mind (or Body)

Any delusion which involves an external force penetrating the subject's mind or body, e.g. rays turn his liver to gold, alien thoughts pierce his skull or are inserted into his mind, hypnotism makes him levitate.

Primary Delusions (Delusional Perceptions)

These are based on sensory experiences (delusional perceptions) in which a subject suddenly becomes convinced that a particular set of events has a special meaning (of a highly specific kind – see text). It frequently follows a delusional mood.

Sexual Delusions

Any delusion with sexual content, e.g. fantasy lover, sex changing, etc.

Morbid Jealousy

The subject believes his partner is being unfaithful.

Delusions of Pregnancy

The subject thinks she is pregnant although the circumstances make it clear that she cannot possibly be. For example, one subject was a widow, had not had intercourse for several years, was well past the menopause, but was convinced she had been pregnant for two years.

Delusions of Guilt

This symptom appears to be grounded in a depressed mood. The subject feels he has committed a crime, or sinned greatly, or has brought ruin to his family or on the world. He may feel he deserves punishment, even death or hell-fire.

Simple Delusions concerning Appearance

The subject has a strong feeling that something is wrong with his appearance. He looks old or ugly or dead, his skin is cracked, his teeth misshapen, his nose too large, or his body crooked, etc. Other people do not notice anything specially wrong but the subject can be reassured only momentarily if at all.

Delusions of Depersonalization or Nihilism

The subject is convinced that he has no head, has a hollow instead of a brain, that he cannot see himself in the mirror, that he has a shadow but no body, does not exist.

Hypochondriacal Delusions

The subject feels that his body is unhealthy, rotten or diseased. If more intense, he feels he has incurable cancer, his bowels are stopped up, his insides are rotting, etc.

Delusions of Catastrophe

The subject believes that the world is about to end, some enormous catastrophe has occurred or will occur, or everything is evil and will be destroyed.

Delusions of Thoughts Being Read

This is usually an explanatory delusion, for example of delusions of reference or misinterpretation, which require some explanation of how other people know so much about the patient's future movements. It may be an elaboration of thought broadcast, thought insertion, auditory hallucinations, delusions of control, delusions of persecution or delusions of influence. It can even occur with expansive delusions (e.g. as an explanation of how Einstein stole the subject's ideas).

Delusion that the Subject Smells

The subject irrationally thinks that he gives off a smell and that others notice it and react accordingly.

The PSE also offered a helpful distinction between delusions of reference and a superficially similar but non-psychotic phenomenon, *simple ideas of reference*:

> In its moderate form, this symptom is indicated by selfconsciousness. The subject cannot help feeling that people take notice of him – in buses, in a restaurant, or in other public places – and that they observe things about him that he would prefer not to be seen. He realizes that this feeling originates within himself and that he is no more noticed than other people, but cannot help the feeling all the same, quite out of proportion to any possible cause ... In its severe form, the subject thinks that people are critical of him, or that they tend to laugh at him. Often he is ashamed of something and cannot help feeling that others are aware of what it is. He realizes that this feeling originates within himself.

Most people have experienced this symptom at one time or another, a typical example being when you enter a room and notice that the people there go quiet, as if they had just been talking about you. This feeling is swiftly followed by the realization that it is probably just your imagination (or at least that it would not be a good idea to mention it). As described in Chapters 2 and 3, in some circumstances, such ideas can become pervasive.

Delusions where there is no component of abnormal significance make up a large group in Wing et al.'s (1974) classification. They include the obvious category of delusions of persecution. A little-known variant of this is the *delusion of assistance*, where patients believe that organizations of the same kind are trying to help them in surreptitious ways. The PSE distinguishes two subcategories of grandiose delusions, *delusions of grandiose ability* and *delusions of grandiose identity*. There are also *religious delusions*, which are often but not necessarily grandiose in nature.

The wilder end of the delusional spectrum is represented in the PSE in a single item for *fantastic delusions*, *delusional memories* and *delusional confabulation*. One reason why these symptoms were grouped together by Wing et al. (1974) may be that they are uncommon and when they are seen they tend to occur together. Some examples of delusional memories are shown in Box 1.4. An example of delusional confabulation is shown in Box 1.5. (For more examples see McKenna, 1994; McKenna, 2007; Shakeel & Docherty, 2015.)

Box 1.4 Examples of Delusional Memories in Patients with Schizophrenia (Author's Own Cases)

A young woman was asked the PSE question 'Have you had any unusual experience or adventures recently?' She replied by describing how she had been swimming a few weeks earlier and her stomach split open and the swimming pool filled with blood.

A male patient believed that he was being tortured by a machine which he had invented as a child. He described how one day in primary school the teacher asked all the children in his class to invent something and bring it to school the next day. He described some of the inventions the other children brought. He brought a prototype of his machine, which the teacher then stole.

A female patient recalled Prince Charles and Princess Diana being present in the delivery room when she was born. She saw no contradiction in the fact that she was approximately the same age as Princess Diana.

During the course of an interview to assess his suitability for transfer to a rehabilitation service, a young male patient described in detail how, some months previously, his brain had been removed from his body and transported to America in a plane. His recall of what happened next was slightly hazy, but he remembered his brain being placed on a wheelchair and transported by limousine to a recording studio where it made a record with a well-known rap star.

An unmarried female patient, who had never travelled outside the county where she was born, believed that she had been married to a series of policemen. Some of these were American and she described how she and one of them had lived in Los Angeles. When asked where in Los Angeles she replied, 'Just off the San Francisco road.' She also described a trip to Mount Everest, where she noticed there was a lot of litter, and a holiday in New York with a friend, during which they went to see Frank Sinatra.

Box 1.5 Delusional Confabulation (Author's Own Case)

The last patient in the previous Box 1.4 had a diagnosis of chronic schizophrenia (although her clinical picture actually conformed reasonably closely to Kraepelin's confabulatory paraphrenia). While she consistently believed that she had lived abroad and been married to a number of different policemen, the details changed from day to day, and she also embellished her accounts as she talked. On one occasion, her account went as follows:

I. How long have you been with him [Marshall, her current boyfriend]?
P. For years.
I. Have you had any boyfriends before?
P. Yes, I've had six. Five of them I married. The first of them was when I was quite a young child.
I. You were married when you were a child?
P. No, he was only a boyfriend.
I. It was the next one?
P. Yes, it was the next one, James.
I. And what happened to James?
P. He died in Vietnam.
I. How did it happen?
P. Well he was an American.
I. What happened then? Did you get married again?
P. Yes, I got married to Jim.
I. Can you tell me a bit about Jim?
P. Well, he was a very nice man, good sense of humour and ... he died out in Vietnam as well.
I. He did?
P. I lost two husbands very quickly.
I. How long were you married to Jim?
P. Only a few months.
I. Well, did you remain unmarried afterwards or did you marry again?
P. I got married again in my early 30s.
I. To who?
P. That was to Alan, I'd known him for years, he was a friend of James and Jim.
I. Do you remember what sort of occupation he had?
P. He was a police officer. He died in Ireland.
I. In Ireland? So what happened in Ireland then?
P. I don't exactly know how he died out there.
I. Where was it in Ireland?
P. In Belfast.
I. Do you remember any of the circumstances?

P. I don't know how Jim died – he was another Jim, before I married Geoff. Well, I know how Geoff died. We'd just gone out to the shops and someone threw a large brick or stone or something and he thought that it had hit me and he collapsed and died. Because I swayed a bit. It only missed me by a fraction. It only just really came by a fraction away.

[Slightly later]

I. What about your next husband?

P. After Geoff it was Marshall.

I. And where does he live?

P. Well, he's got a house in ... he was born in 5 Watford Avenue, Bury St Edmunds 30 years ago when I was only 7. I call him Marshall as a nickname because he's always giving me mars bars. His real name is Dr Paul Black Hadfield ... I've known him since the day he was born. 'Cause I was at Bury police station and his father invited me to come down to the house.

Hypochondriacal delusions in the PSE refer only to beliefs about having a serious illness such as cancer or heart disease. More fanciful beliefs about bodily change or malfunction, for example that one's nose is made of metal, or one's liver has been turned to gold, are rated as fantastic delusions. The PSE also has a category for simple delusions concerning one's appearance, e.g. about one's nose being too large, or one's teeth misshapen, and also the belief that one gives off an offensive smell. Whether or not these latter kinds of beliefs always take the form of delusions is a question that is considered in depth in Chapters 2 and 3.

A third class of delusions in the PSE share the feature that they appear to be secondary to another form of psychopathology. These include *delusions of sin, guilt and worthlessness*, whose content seems obviously related to depressed mood. Sometimes this type of delusion takes on spectacular proportions: in Cotard's syndrome patients state that they are the worst sinner in the world, their bowels are stopped up or rotting, they have no body, they do not exist, they are dead, or alternatively cannot die and are doomed to walk the Earth for eternity. Generations of psychiatrists have wondered whether the Cotard syndrome might not be a delusional elaboration of the symptom of depersonalization/derealization (see Enoch et al., 1967; Enoch & Ball, 2001) where patients feel as if their own body and/or their surroundings are unreal, with the 'as if' indicating that they know that that this not really the case. Accordingly, the PSE has an item for *delusions of depersonalization*.

Wing et al. (1974) dispensed altogether with another time-honoured usage of the term secondary delusions, to describe beliefs that seem clearly to be based on another psychotic symptom. Examples here include patients who believe they have a radio transmitter in their head because of the experience that their thoughts are available to all and sundry, or that the voices they hear are caused by people being inside their body. Instead, the PSE uses the term *delusional explanations* for such symptoms.

What the PSE calls *delusions of control* is essentially the same symptom that Bleuler (1911) identified as ideas of influence and Schneider (1958) called somatic passivity. Here patients feel that they are under the force or power of some external agency which makes them move their arms or legs, talks using their mouth, etc. This symptom may also be a delusional explanation: as part of his general theory that schizophrenic symptoms are due to a failure of monitoring (see Chapter 5), Frith (1992) argued that there is sometimes a failure to label one's own movements as self-generated. This would give rise to a compelling sensation that one's movements were not one's own, which could then serve as the basis for a belief about being controlled by alien forces.

Finally, almost in passing, Wing et al. (1974) recognized the occurrence of what they called *partial or partially held delusions*. These refer to beliefs that are expressed with doubt, as a possibility which the subject is prepared to entertain but is not certain about. This might be because the delusion has not yet fully formed, or alternatively it might have been held with full conviction previously but not at the time of rating (for example, as a result of treatment). This may or may not have been an attempt to update Jaspers' (1959) argument that fixity of conviction is a poor criterion for judging whether a belief is delusional, but in any case it corresponds to clinical reality.

Conclusion: So What Are Delusions?

After a century of description and redescription, plus a certain amount of healthy debate, the outlook for delusions does not seem nearly as gloomy as David (1999) portrayed it at the beginning of this chapter. It may still not be possible to define delusions in a way that captures them in their endlessly varying forms, while at the same time excluding the forms of normal belief they can be confused with, but there does seem to have been some progress in delineating their characteristic features.

One feature of delusions that emerges strongly is just how extraordinary a phenomenon they are. Rather than representing some kind of exaggeration of the kinds of unrealistic thinking and flights of fancy we are all prone to from time to time, they seem not to resemble normal beliefs very much at all. Their point of departure is the impossible (or perhaps more accurately the nearly impossible), and from there they ascend to dizzying heights of bizarreness and ludicrousness, coming in some cases to violate common sense at its most elementary. In this sense delusions truly are un-understandable.

A second feature of delusions, one that is so obvious that it is often overlooked, is that they are by and large directed to only one relatively small area of the person's beliefs, those about him- or herself. Deluded patients typically believe that they, not other people, are being conspired against, or are suddenly very important, or are undergoing disturbing bodily changes, etc. Occasionally the belief may instead involve people the patient is close to, the obvious example here being the Capgras syndrome, where the patient believes one or more of his or her relatives have been replaced by impostors (see Chapter 7). However, delusions that concern the world at large seem to be unusual – Kraepelin (1913a) described a patient who believed that Christ had been crucified in Germany, and another who invented fictitious life-stories for his fellow patients, and there is an example of a fantastic delusion in the PSE of a belief that England's coast was melting – but the suspicion is that the occurrence of this type of delusions is mostly restricted to very florid delusional states.

As brought into sharp focus by the dispute between Jaspers and Schneider, it seems difficult to avoid the conclusion that there is a broad division within the category of delusions. On the one hand there is a class of delusions, which includes delusions of reference and misinterpretation, and also delusional mood and the rare delusional perception, which have in common that the patient erroneously attributes significance to neutral events going on around him or her. On the other, there is the familiar range of persecutory, grandiose, hypochondriacal and other beliefs which, as far as one can tell, do not contain any intrinsic element of abnormal significance. There is no agreed-on name for this latter class of delusions – 'delusional ideas' seems too vague and Schneider's term 'delusional intuitions' now sounds quaint – so from now on they will be referred to as *propositional delusions* (based on the dictionary definition of a proposition as a statement that expresses a judgement or opinion, or is asserted to be true). How these two forms of delusions relate to each other will be a theme that crops up repeatedly throughout this book.

It also appears that there might be a significant division within the category of propositional delusions itself. Some such beliefs are self-contained and sometimes appear as it were out of nowhere (although they can also grow out of referential delusions). Others, however, while being delusions in every sense of the term, draw their content from other symptoms such as pathologically altered mood or auditory hallucinations. The idea of delusions being secondary or explanatory has had an enormous impact on thinking about the symptom, featuring in one of the earliest experimental psychological theories (see Chapter 5) all the way through to contemporary approaches (see Chapter 7 and Chapter 8).

When Is a Delusion Not a Delusion?

Focusing on beliefs that everyone would agree are delusional, as was done in Chapter 1, can tell us quite a lot about their defining characteristics and perhaps even say something about their underlying nature. However this approach is silent on another question, of whether there are other forms of pathological belief, and if so how these might be related to delusions. Also left unanswered is the question of the status of unusual beliefs that are seen in the non-mentally ill population, and whether or not these are related to delusions. The first of these issues turns out to be non-trivial and is the subject of this chapter. Discussion of the second, that of minority and idiosyncratic beliefs in the non-psychotic population, is postponed to Chapter 4.

The outstanding, even notorious, example of a belief that is pathological but not considered to be delusional is the overvalued idea. This clinical construct has been in existence for over a century, during which time it has been a constant thorn in the side of those who prefer their definitions of delusions to be simple. Although it often seems to lead a shady existence on the fringes of psychiatry, the need for such a category of abnormal belief has been argued for several times over the years, not least by Jaspers (1959). Rather more frequently, however, the reaction has been one of bland denial that there is any case to answer.

Another class of belief that falls squarely into the category of pathological but only uncomfortably regarded as delusional are the ideas of hopelessness, self-depreciation and self-blame that are seen in major depression. Clearly, depressed patients who are convinced that they are never going to get better despite having recovered from numerous previous similar episodes, and believe they are a burden on their families who would be better off without them, are labouring under some form of false belief. However, most people would be reluctant to place such ideas in the same category as those of Kraepelin's patient in the previous chapter who wrongly believed that her husband was dead and that it was her fault. Exactly the same issues arise in mania, where patients with milder forms of the illness show boundless confidence and have inflated ideas about their abilities and future prospects. Despite the fact that clinicians encounter these ideas on a regular basis, they have been subject to very little scrutiny and they never seem to have acquired a universally accepted formal psychopathological name. In this chapter they are referred to rather clumsily as the unfounded ideas of major affective disorder.

The third form of non-delusional abnormal belief that needs to be considered seems at first sight surprising, since it concerns obsessions. Medical students the world over are taught that, although patients with obsessive-compulsive disorder find themselves forced to think unpleasant and distressing thoughts, they recognize that the ideas are not true. Later, those medical students who go on to become psychiatrists learn that some patients are distinctly ambivalent in their attitude to their obsessions, and there are even some who deny altogether that their ideas are irrational. How patients who show this phenomenon should be regarded might be thought to be a matter of only academic interest. However, it has recently acquired some importance, as psychiatry has found itself wrestling with the problem of how to classify not only patients who do not doubt their obsessions, but also those with certain other non-psychotic disorders where the ideas sometimes seem to be held with full delusional intensity (above all body dysmorphic disorder, see Chapter 3).

Overvalued Ideas

In the early 1980s the author of this book decided to carry out a PSE, which he had just learnt how to do, on a patient with morbid jealousy, a man who was convinced his wife was being unfaithful. He was confident that the detailed questioning of the interview would reveal not only a central delusion of infidelity but also a supporting network of delusions of reference and misinterpretation. After all, this was what such patients were supposed to show according to the literature on what was then variously referred to as paranoia, paranoid state and paranoid psychosis, which included a jealous subtype. To this author's surprise, while the patient was completely convinced that his wife was having extramarital sex indiscriminately, he denied all other symptoms. He did not believe that people were talking about his wife's infidelity, or that there were references to it on the TV, or that her lovers were leaving secret messages for her, or anything of the kind. He did think he could detect signs of his wife's sexual activity from the state of her underwear, which he checked constantly, but this seemed to be understandable as the kind of wrong conclusion that anyone who was deliberately searching for scraps of confirmatory evidence might easily come to.

This was the author's introduction to the murky world of the overvalued idea, the tradition that there exists a form of abnormal belief with qualities that set it apart from delusions, even if it is difficult to say exactly why. The term had been introduced by Wernicke at the beginning of the twentieth century (Wernicke, 1906), who defined it as a solitary abnormal belief that came to dominate an individual's actions to a morbid degree. Unlike obsessions, overvalued ideas were viewed as normal by the patient; '[i]ndeed patients see in them expressions of their very being'. Their development could often be traced to an event that aroused strong emotions of a negative kind, for example being left out of a will, the suicide of a friend, the death of one's husband, a wife's comment about sniffing tobacco, witnessing a person being deloused and perhaps most characteristically receiving an official judgement that was perceived to be unfair. Although the ideas often developed in individuals without any other signs of psychopathology, they could also be the first sign of psychosis or a symptom of melancholia or general paralysis (i.e. neurosyphilis).

The first case Wernicke described was of a 61-year-old man who came to psychiatric attention when he had an altercation with two men outside his flat. The police were called and the upshot was that he was forcibly removed to a mental hospital. No psychotic symptoms were found and he was quickly discharged. However, similar incidents continued to occur, leading to more admissions. It emerged that the patient believed that one of the two men involved in the original dispute, who he was acquainted with, had said to the other something along the lines of 'Look, there is the scoundrel who abandoned the girl that time.' The patient took this to be a reference to the fact that he had previously proposed to the daughter of a wine trader, but then broke off the engagement when he found out that her father was in financial difficulties. He considered that the escalating harassment he was experiencing all went back to this acquaintance, who had told other people the story and had also instigated the police to observe him on the grounds of alleged mental illness. The patient ended up hospitalized continuously for four years; he showed no referential ideas or other signs of mental illness during his stay, but he did not want to leave because he was convinced the harassment would start up again.

Wernicke's second case was different, and foreshadowed some of the problems that would dog the overvalued idea in years to come. It concerned an unmarried female schoolteacher of around 40 who started to believe that a male colleague was in love with her. This caused her such difficulties that she ultimately had to leave her job. Unlike the previous patient, referentiality was a prominent part of the clinical picture, and this may well have gone beyond what could be construed just as simple ideas of reference. She repeatedly found herself in apparently coincidental meetings with the male colleague, and noticed that other members of staff talked conspicuously about him; even her pupils seemed to be dropping hints about the matter. A decisive feature for Wernicke was the fact that, despite having been declared incurably insane at one point, she eventually improved dramatically and returned to work in another job. Nevertheless, she remained permanently estranged from her family, who she believed deserved some of the blame for her losing the love of her life.

Despite being contemporaries of Wernicke, Kraepelin and Bleuler had very little to say about overvalued ideas. Kraepelin seems not to have used the term, and Bleuler (1924) expressed doubt about whether the symptom existed. Even so, both authors found themselves grappling with the problem of patients who showed similar features to Wernicke's first case. Kraepelin (1905) gave a detailed description of one such patient (see Box 2.1), and argued that the presentation was simply a 'secondary form' of paranoia. Later, however, he (Kraepelin, 1913b) changed his mind and excluded it from this category, citing among other things the fact that the belief seemed to have its basis in external events rather than arising from than internal causes.

Box 2.1 The Querulous Paranoid State (Kraepelin, 1905)

A master tailor, who had previously been declared bankrupt, again fell into debt and, in the course of trying to prevent a creditor and a bailiff removing his furniture, locked both of them up in his house while he lodged a complaint in court. As a consequence of this he was found guilty of false imprisonment.

A short, humorously treated account of the affair appeared in a newspaper, which contained inaccuracies. The patient wrote a correction, only part of which was printed. A further enraged letter to the editor was responded to by publication of a full report of the proceedings, in which the words 'master tailor' were printed in large type. The patient took exception to this and brought three legal actions against the newspaper. These actions were all rejected in the courts. The patient then set in motion a series of appeals to higher and higher courts, eventually petitioning the Ministry of Justice, the Ministry of State, the Grand Duke and the Emperor. After all these measures failed he tried the experiment of complaining to the heads of the courts and appealing to the public, and was considering proposing disciplinary proceedings against the Public Prosecutor.

The all-consuming nature of the patient's preoccupation was well-illustrated in the following passage:

> The innumerable petitions which the patient has drawn up in the course of the last few years, chiefly at night, are exceedingly long-winded, and always allege the same thing in a rather disconnected manner. In their form and mode of expression they incline to the legal document, beginning

with 'Concerning', going on throughout with 'evidence' and concluding with 'grounds'. They abound in half or wholly misunderstood professional expressions and paragraphs of totally different laws. Often they are careless and appear to have been written under excitement, contain numerous notes of exclamation and interrogation, even in the middle of a sentence; one or more underlinings, some in red or blue pencil; marginal notes and addenda, so that every available space is made use of. Many of the petitions are written on the backs of judgements and refusals of other courts.

On mental state examination, the patient was coherent and was able to give a clear account of events. On the subject of his court actions he expressed himself volubly and showed increased self-confidence and superiority, plus a certain satisfaction and readiness for battle. He was also exceedingly touchy – if pressed on whether he might have been mistaken in his interpretation of events, he immediately became mistrustful and raised the suspicion that the interviewer supported his opponents. He was never at a loss for an answer to objections, which he justified by quoting minutiae of the law; in prolonged conversation a wearisome diffuseness crept into his narrative. It seemed that an attorney involved in the patient's original bankruptcy proceedings was the original source of his problems. Because of this, the clerk did not draw up the accusation properly; the public prosecutor gained an erroneous impression from it; and the judges of several courts did not want to reverse verdicts once agreed to; and as a body they were prejudiced. He believed that the whole system of law had been obstructed via a conspiracy involving Freemasons and also Jewish financiers, who supported the newspaper that wrote about him. Additionally, the press was involved, as they were associated with the attorney in question.

As a result of his incessant pestering of the authorities, the patient was eventually pronounced to be mentally deranged, against which he adopted every possible legal means of redress. Meanwhile he continued to carry on his business, and apart from writing innumerable petitions, did not appear strange or troublesome. He had brought his family almost to the brink of ruin, but in spite of all the setbacks he remained optimistic about the outcome of his case.

Bleuler (1911) expressed his views rather more succinctly:

We find numerous transitions from simply unbearable people to the paranoid litigants with marked delusions. The best solution perhaps is to draw a line somewhere in the middle of the scale and place the half that do not have real delusions there and count the others as paranoid.

In contrast to Kraepelin and Bleuler, Jaspers (1959) wholeheartedly embraced the concept of the overvalued idea. For him it was one of the most important categories of delusion-like ideas, beliefs that needed to be distinguished from delusions proper (others included the delusions of mania and depression and what he called transient deceptions due to false perception). Unlike delusions, which were the manifestations of a new process irrupting into the individual's life, an overvalued idea was, he argued, the result of an interaction between the individual and his experience which brought a focus to the patient's life, albeit a pathological one – it was as it were a 'hypertrophy' of an already abnormal personality in reaction to adverse events.

Psychopathologically, rather than being un-understandable, the overvalued idea was fundamentally no different to the kinds of passionate political, religious or ethical conviction held by many healthy people. As well as the by now paradigmatic querulous paranoid state, Jaspers (1959) considered that a proportion of patients with morbid jealousy also showed overvalued ideas, as well as some cranky inventors and world reformers.

Jaspers' views on understandability versus un-understandability and process versus personality development enjoyed great influence in mid-twentieth century British and

European psychiatry, but started to fall out of fashion from the 1970s. Over roughly the same period, the overvalued idea made the transition into a much looser usage, as a term which referred to false beliefs that the clinician did not feel were held with the degree of full conviction necessary for delusions – in other words as a synonym for partial delusions (see Chapter 1). This position became official in 1980 when DSM-III defined an overvalued idea as 'an unreasonable and sustained belief that is maintained with less than delusional intensity (i.e. the person is able to acknowledge the possibility that the belief may or may not be true)'.

The overvalued idea was not to prove quite so easy to dispose of, however. The problem was the existence of certain disorders which were characterised by a range of presentations that were difficult to fully characterize without resorting to something resembling the concept. One of these was morbid jealousy, which encompassed everything from merely over-possessive individuals to patients who held a delusion of infidelity in the context of an obviously psychotic illness with other delusions, hallucinations, etc. In between were patients – like the one described earlier in this chapter – who showed a preoccupying belief that their partner was being unfaithful in the apparent absence of other symptoms, variously referred to in the literature as jealous monomania, obsessive jealousy or the jealousy reaction of abnormal persons (Cobb, 1979). Another example was hypochondriasis: Merskey (1979) commented that between the excessive health consciousness that characterized many otherwise psychiatrically healthy individuals and the delusions of illness and bodily malfunction seen in major depression and schizophrenia, from time to time one encountered patients for whom pure hypochondriasis seemed the only applicable term:

> These patients show excessive concern with bodily function, a failure to respond to sympathetic management and reassurance by relinquishing their complaint, a marked fear of the occurrence of physical disease and a continuing or markedly recurring belief that they have got a disease. They show dependence on medical personnel and often are dissatisfied with them. A pattern of cultivated meticulous valetudinarianism may be prominent together with detailed ordering of the smallest items of daily life in terms of health and illness with cupboards overflowing with laxatives and home remedies, punctilious compliance with dietary fads, etc.

Eventually, the present author (McKenna, 1984), prompted by his own experience with the aforesaid patient with morbid jealousy (who ultimately murdered his wife), and having also seen a case of querulous paranoia, not to mention several with hypochondriasis, made the connection with the tradition of the overvalued idea and wrote a review article on the topic. This made the point that all three disorders could sometimes occur in an isolated form, without other symptoms suggestive of schizophrenia or major depression being present. The phenomenology of the belief, it was suggested (only partly tongue-in-cheek), was characterized by non-delusional conviction, non-obsessional preoccupation and non-phobic fear. A further notable feature was the determined and consistent way in which the patients acted on their beliefs.

The article also made a case that the central feature of some other disorders was an overvalued idea. The classic example here was anorexia nervosa where, despite the fact that patients adamantly believe they are overweight – to the extent that they not infrequently starve themselves to death – use of the term delusion was (and still is) studiously avoided. Something else that seemed like it might fit into the same category was dysmorphophobia, or as it is now known, body dysmorphic disorder. The nosological status of this disorder was very unclear at the time, as witnessed by articles with titles like 'Dysmorphophobia: symptom or disease' (Andreasen & Bardach, 1977). Since then interest has increased exponentially, and the question of whether these patients are deluded or not deluded is currently the subject of an important debate (see Chapter 3).

A third suggested candidate for a disorder with an overvalued idea was erotomania. Although Wernicke's (1900) second patient had this diagnosis, her case was less than convincing as she had widespread referential ideas that may well have been delusional in nature. However, de Clérambault (1942, see also Baruk, 1959), whose name has become synonymous with the disorder, also felt that erotomania showed features that set it apart from other delusional states. Rather than being a gradually discovered explanation for mysterious events, he argued, the belief in erotomania had a 'passionate' or 'hypersthenic' quality from the outset, which led the patient to relentlessly pursue the person they believed was in love with them. Unfortunately, de Clérambault's five cases of 'pure' erotomania (as described in Signer, 1991) were no more convincing than Wernicke's: one believed that a whole series of military officers and King George V were secretly communicating their romantic interest in her and that all London knew about the affair. Another showed formal thought disorder, and a third additionally had persecutory delusions.

Nevertheless, there is some reason to believe that cases of erotomania where the central belief shows the hallmarks of an overvalued idea may also exist. Mullen et al. (2000) described a form of the disorder which often emerged in an individual with pre-existing personality vulnerabilities such as self-consciousness, stubbornness and a tendency to take remarks the wrong way, and once established, became the organizing principle of the person's life. Although they stated that the belief was often of delusional intensity, they also noted that on other matters the individual remained as clear thinking, orderly and rational as before they became ill. The central belief did not even have to be a conviction that a person was in love with the patient; patients with what they termed pathologically infatuations (also known as borderline erotomania) persistently pursued the object of their affections but made no strong claims that their love was reciprocated. One of Mullen et al.'s cases of this type is reproduced in Box 2.2.

Box 2.2 Borderline Erotomania or Pathological Infatuation (Mullen et al., 2000)

Ms L, a female aged 47, was the youngest of four children. On leaving school she obtained a job as an accounts clerk, which she had retained until a year previously. Her husband was her first and only boyfriend. Ms L was always painfully shy and self-conscious. She reported frequently feeling that people looked at her and laughed at her behind her back. At work she was occasionally overwhelmed by suspicions that others were ganging up on her and talking about her. She avoided social contacts outside the family. She was a well-organized individual but had no obsessional or phobic symptoms.

Four years previously she had come to 'realize' that a senior partner in the firm for which she worked entertained romantic feelings about her. She had always admired him and considered him a gentle and concerned individual. Her preoccupations with this man increased markedly after the sudden death of a younger brother who had been the person with whom she had had the closest relationship. The love crystallized following an incident when the object of her affections spoke to her one morning about the weather and the prospects for the upcoming ski season. It was this she claimed made her realize that he reciprocated her affection. She said 'I knew this meant he had strong feelings for me, because usually I am completely ignored. No one chats to me. They think I'm not intelligent enough'.

Over the next few months she felt that he expressed his love in a variety of roundabout ways: clothes that he wore, the way he nodded a greeting, and the occasional exchanged good morning. It was not, she said, so much what he said but the tone of voice and the way he said it. She became interested in her appearance for the first time in many years, took up aerobics, lost 10 kg and began colouring her hair.

The object of her attentions, in a victim impact statement, said he had been aware for some years that she was infatuated with him, but this was entirely one sided and had never been encouraged. He had tried to ignore it but it became, in the last three years, increasingly intrusive. She would follow him; turn up unexpectedly; stand next to his car after work, awaiting his departure; write notes to him and phone him both at work and at home. He arranged for her to be made redundant to prevent continuing harassment at work.

Eight months prior to the admission, Ms L, while trailing the object of her affections, observed him to meet and have a drink with a senior secretary from the firm's office. Over the next week she tailed both this lady and the object of her affections. She became convinced that he was having an affair with this woman. She found herself troubled by intrusive images of her would-be lover in the arms of this other woman. She became increasingly distressed and angry. She made a number of accusatory phone calls to the object of her affections, his wife and the secretary she supposed to have stolen his affections from her. At one point she attempted to throw herself in front of his car. She caused a major incident at his place of work by accusing him in front of a number of colleagues of having an affair and having deserted her. At this time she began to develop signs of depression with sleep disturbance, loss of appetite, self-denigratory ruminations and suicidal thoughts. Immediately prior to her admission she confronted the object of her affections with a rifle she had taken from her husband's gun cupboard. He claims she pointed it at him and threatened him, although she denies actually directing the gun at him. She left to return home, where she attempted to stab herself through the heart and in fact succeeded in inflicting a serious chest wound.

On admission she acknowledged that she was still preoccupied by thoughts of her supposed lover. She believed that there would still be a reconciliation between them because he remained in love with her and she returned his affection. She acknowledged that she was still plagued by jealousy and that vivid images would intrude into her consciousness of him having intercourse with her supposed rival. She claimed no longer to be actively suicidal because she recognized that eventually this hiccup in their relationship would be sorted out and they would have a future together. She was commenced on both antidepressants and 6 mg of pimozide and over the subsequent four weeks, the intensity of her preoccupations with this supposed beloved gradually decreased. She came to recognize that the relationship was now over and there was no future, given what had occurred. She still retained the belief that he had returned her affections, although she accepted that she may have been overhopeful in her expectations for the relationship.

The stage was now set for a further expansion of the concept of the overvalued idea by Veale (2002). He argued that it had been a mistake all along to think of overvalued ideas in terms of concepts like degree of conviction and presence or absence of insight. Instead, he proposed that the overvalued idea occupied a different conceptual space altogether, that of Beck's (1979) 'personal domain'. An individual's personal domain concerns what he or she values about him- or herself, the animate and inanimate objects that he or she has an emotional investment in, such as his family, friends and possessions. Overvalued ideas arose when one of these values became dominant and idealized within the personal domain. Conversely, if a particular value was not part of an individual's personal domain, an overvalued idea could not develop: a person may believe that they are overweight or their nose is

Table 2.1 Some Additional Disorders Where the Central Psychopathology Has Been Proposed to Be an Overvalued Idea

Disorder	Value(s) That Have Become Idealized and/or Dominant	Typical Beliefs
Anorexia nervosa	Self-control especially of weight and shape, and in some patients perfectionism, define the identity of the person. Even in the face of overwhelming evidence that others do not think they are fat or defective, they are still more concerned with their own values than any external standard.	'I feel I'm fat'
Body dysmorphic disorder	Appearance, and in some cases perfectionism and being socially accepted. As with anorexia nervosa, they are more concerned with their own values than any external standard.	'My nose is crooked and ugly'
Gender dysphoria	Correct gender; sexual characteristics are no longer part of the self.	'I feel I am the wrong sex'
Pseudocyesis	Children are at the centre of personal domain	'I feel pregnant'
Compulsive hoarding	Self as a custodian or caretaker; the individual's belongings have become of paramount importance and define one's identity	'I think my jewellery is lost'
Apotemnophilia	Self viewed as a deformed object; one or more limbs have become placed far away from the centre of a personal domain	'My limb does not belong to me. I need it to be amputated to be comfortable'

Note: Veale also included social phobia, making the argument that patients at the severe end of the spectrum of this disorder often hold beliefs with near delusional certainty about what others are thinking.
Source: Veale, D. (2002). Over-valued ideas: a conceptual analysis. Behaviour Research and Therapy, 40, 383–400.

too big, but if they do not place much value on the importance of appearance, this will never convert into anorexia nervosa or body dysmorphic disorder.

This conceptualization led Veale (2002) to propose that overvalued ideas are the common feature of a considerably wider range of disorders than previously thought. A partial list of the disorders he included is shown in Table 2.1; notable inclusions are gender dysphoria, compulsive hoarding and pseudocyesis. In gender dysphoria, he argued, the idealized value is being of the opposite gender, and in compulsive hoarding it is the individual's possessions that assume overriding importance. Women with pseudocyesis believe themselves to be pregnant when they are not, reflecting the enormous emotional investment they have in having children. It is worth noting that there is little or no psychiatric understanding of any of these disorders, either from the standpoint of nosology or in terms of their putative psychopathological basis.

The last disorder listed in Table 2.1 has to be among the strangest in psychiatry. Apotemnophilia or body integrity identity disorder is a thankfully rare condition where an individual develops an overwhelming wish to have one or more limbs amputated. This leads him or her to try and persuade surgeons to operate to remove a limb, or in some cases self-amputation is attempted. The scanty available information (Blom et al., 2012; First, 2005; First & Fisher, 2012) suggests that the disorder usually has its onset in childhood or adolescence and that only a minority of patients have associated psychiatric disorders. Although not sexually motivated in the majority of cases, the disorder otherwise seems to share several key features with gender dysphoria, as First (2005) noted.

Something that Veale (2002) did not include but might represent yet another example of a disorder with an overvalued idea, at least in some cases, is the olfactory reference syndrome, currently classified as a subtype of delusional disorder (see Chapter 3). These patients become convinced that they give off an offensive smell which others notice, and they engage excessively in behaviours such as showering, changing their underwear and using perfumes and deodorants. Begum and McKenna (2011) carried out a systematic review of cases reported in the world literature, excluding those which showed – or later developed – evidence of schizophrenia, major depression or bipolar disorder. They found that while some of the patients were described as holding the belief that they smelt with unwavering conviction, in slightly less than half there were statements such as, 'admitted that his preoccupations about the odour were excessive and unreasonable'; 'the thoughts were ego-dystonic'; 'oscillated between fear and conviction'; and 'could be persuaded to some extent that she did not smell'. They also found that only a minority of the patients were actually able to smell the smell they believed they were giving off, and even then often only intermittently. Referential thinking, in contrast, was very frequent – the patients described people around them frowning, making remarks, opening windows, getting off buses and trains when the patient got on, and so on. However, while these ideas were often pervasive and at times farfetched, they never seemed to take a clearly delusional form, such as the smell being referred to by means of special signs or being alluded to on television.

Unfounded Ideas in Major Affective Disorder

The description of this phenomenon goes back to well before the time of Kraepelin and Bleuler, but it seems only right to start with the former author, who, as well as identifying schizophrenia, was the first to properly define the category of major affective disorder. Describing 'melancholia simplex', that is depressive states without psychotic symptoms or stupor, he (Kraepelin, 1913b) noted how the patients viewed their past and future in a uniformly dim light: they felt that they were worthless and no longer of any use, their life appeared pointless to them, and they considered themselves superfluous in the world. In more severe forms of illness, the ideas would become first more and more remote from reality – patients would state that they had not taken good care of their children, had not paid their bills punctually, had been dishonest about their taxes – and then frankly delusional – that they had committed perjury, offended a highly placed person without knowing it, committed incest, set fire to their house, etc.

In much the same way, patients with hypomania, Kraepelin's mildest form of mania, would say things like they were musically gifted, had written poetry, or were more intelligent than anyone else, often in a half-joking or boastful way. Once again these ideas would then give way by degrees to frank delusions in more severe cases, such as of being a millionaire, having invented non-existent devices and so on.

Almost all of what has been written subsequently about these ideas has concerned depression, and the line taken has always been the same, that they shade inexorably into depressive delusions. A good example is the detailed account of 61 patients with melancholia carried out in 1934 by the British psychiatrist, Lewis (1934) (his definition of melancholia corresponds closely to the modern concept of major depression). He found 27 who had prominent ideas of self-reproach and self-accusation. Their ideas ranged from simply expressing the view that they had been selfish, had let everyone down, had neglected their children or had betrayed a trust, to the most abject delusions, for example that they were the wickedest person in the world, or that they had plotted to bring about their husband's death through consumption, or that by eating they were causing other people to starve.

Hypochondriacal ideas were also common, being seen in 25 of the patients. The ideas here often centred on the bowels and once again encompassed the kind of concerns expressed by many healthy people, through to more obviously pathological ideas that they could not digest their food, to in the most severe examples a complete denial of having any abdominal viscera.

Something that Lewis (1934) did not describe but which can also occur is a transition from unfounded ideas to delusions in the same patient. Most clinicians will have seen patients who initially present with vague complaints about their bowels, without any clear diagnosis, but then over a period of days or weeks go on to develop a picture of psychotic major depression with the earlier ideas transforming into full-blown hypochondriacal delusions.

The only other systematic investigation into the phenomenon of non-delusional depressive ideas that appears to exist is Beck's (1967) description of what he called cognitive distortions. As with Lewis, his case material consisted of patients he was treating, most or all of whom would have met current criteria for major depression or bipolar depression based on a long list of additional symptoms that they were required to show. His analysis was based on the patients' spontaneous reports about their thoughts and feelings during therapy, and also the notes that many of the patients themselves made between sessions.

Beck (1967) found that a particular style of thinking recurred in his patients and showed itself in various ways, including low self-regard, ideas of deprivation (both emotional and material), self-criticism and self-blame, the perception of problems and duties as overwhelming, self-injunctions to do things, and escapist and suicidal wishes. His examples are reproduced in Box 2.3. He observed that such 'depressive cognitions' were often triggered in situations that touched on the patients' preoccupations, even if only in a remote or trivial way. For example, if a passer-by did not smile at one patient, he would think he was inferior. Another patient had the thought she was a bad mother whenever she saw another woman with a child. However, the thoughts could also occur independently of the external situation, in the form of long, uninterrupted sequences of free associations.

Box 2.3 Beck on Depressive Cognitions (Reproduced with permission from Beck, 1967)

Low Self-Regard

This generally consisted of an unrealistic downgrading of themselves in areas that were of particular importance to the patients. A brilliant academician questioned his basic intelligence, an attractive society woman insisted she had become repulsive-looking, and a successful businessman believed he had no real business acumen and was headed for bankruptcy. In making these self-appraisals, the depressed patient was prone to magnify any failure or defects and to minimize or ignore any favorable characteristics. A common feature of many of the self-evaluations was the unfavorable comparison with other people, particularly those in his own social or occupational group. Almost uniformly, in making his comparisons, the depressed patient rated himself as inferior. He regarded himself as less intelligent, less productive, less attractive, less financially secure, or less successful as a spouse or parent than those in his comparison group.

Ideas of Deprivation

These ideas were noted in the patient's verbalized thoughts that he is alone, unwanted, and unlovable, often in the face of overt demonstrations of friendship and affection. The sense of deprivation was also applied to material possessions, despite obvious contrary evidence.

Self-Criticisms and Self-Blame

The self-criticisms, just as the low self-evaluations, were usually applied to those specific attributes or behaviors most highly valued by the individual. A depressed woman, for example, condemned herself for not having breakfast ready for her husband. She reported a sexual affair with one of his colleagues, however, without any evidence of regret, self-criticism, or guilt. Competence as a housewife was one of her expectations of herself but marital fidelity was not. The patients' tendency to blame themselves for their mistakes or shortcomings generally had no logical basis. This was demonstrated by a housewife who took her children on a picnic. When a thunderstorm suddenly appeared, she blamed herself for not having picked a better day.

Overwhelming Problems and Duties

The patients consistently magnified problems or responsibilities that they considered minor or insignificant when not depressed. A depressed housewife, confronted with the necessity of sewing name tags on her children's clothes in preparation for camp, perceived this as a gigantic undertaking that would take weeks to complete. When she finally got to work at it she finished in less than a day.

Self-commands and Injunctions

These cognitions consisted of constant nagging or prodding to do things. The prodding would persist even when it was impractical, undesirable, or impossible for the person to implement these self-instructions. The 'shoulds' and 'musts' were often applied to an enormous range of activities, many of which were mutually exclusive. A housewife reported that in a period of a few minutes, she had compelling thoughts to clean the house, to lose some weight, to visit a sick friend, to be a den mother, to get a full-time job, to plan the week's menus, to return to college for a degree, to spend more time with her children, to take a memory course, to be more active in women's organizations, and to start putting away her family's winter clothes.

Escapist and Suicidal Wishes

Thoughts about escaping from the problems of life were frequent among all the patients. Some had daydreams of being a hobo, or of going to a tropical paradise. It was unusual, however, that evading the tasks brought any relief. Even when a temporary respite was taken on the advice of the psychiatrist, the patients were prone to blame themselves for shirking responsibilities. The desire to escape seemed to be related to the patients' viewing themselves at an impasse. They not only saw themselves as incapable, incompetent, and helpless, but they also saw their tasks as ponderous and formidable. Their response was a wish to withdraw from the 'unsolvable' problems. Several patients spent considerable time in bed; some hiding under the covers. Suicidal preoccupations seemed similarly related to the patient's conceptualization of his situation as untenable or hopeless. He believed he could not tolerate a continuation of his suffering, and he could see no solution to the problem: The psychiatrist could not help him, his symptoms could not be alleviated, and his problems could not be solved.

Beck (1967) also found that depressive cognitions showed certain formal characteristics. One of these was that they arose without any reflection or reasoning: for example, a patient observed that when he was in a situation where someone else was receiving praise he would automatically have the thought, 'I'm nobody ... I'm not good enough'. Later he would reflect on this and realize it was an inappropriate reaction. The thoughts also had an involuntary quality; they would keep occurring even if the patients resolved to stop having them or tried to ward them off. Additionally, they seemed plausible to the patients, who tended to accept them uncritically and often with a strong emotional reaction; it required considerable experience with having the thoughts to be able to see them as distortions. Finally, Beck noted a characteristic stereotyped or perseverative quality: the same type of cognition would be evoked in a wide range of different settings. Some of his patients were even able to anticipate the kinds of depressive thoughts that would occur in certain specific situations and would prepare themselves in advance to make a more realistic judgement of them.

There is a certain amount of re-invention of the wheel in Beck's descriptions, but at the same time there is no doubt that his account has more phenomenological depth than just about anything else that has been written. In particular, he identified depressive unfounded ideas as emerging spontaneously and effortlessly and carrying with them an immediate feeling of being true. In other words they appear to be unmediated, in the same way that Jaspers argued delusions are (see Chapter 1). Unlike delusions, however, patients are able to some extent to distance themselves from the ideas, being able to remonstrate with themselves about them, avoiding situations that provoke them, and most importantly for Beck, being able to be brought round to seeing them as distortions by a therapist.

Depressive cognitions formed the foundation of Beck's development of cognitive therapy, which was to make him as close to world famous as it is possible to get in psychiatry. As he did so, he repeatedly took the position that the ideas were not just present during depressive episodes but represented an enduring aspect of the psychological make-up of individuals are who were prone to develop the disorder (e.g. Beck, 1967, 2008; Kovacs & Beck, 1978). Here, however, he seems to be wrong: Coyne (1989) reviewed the evidence from 10 studies of depressive cognitions in patients who had recovered from a depressive episode. All but one found that the cognitions had returned to levels similar or close to those of controls. The only exception was a study that used less stringent criteria for remission than the other studies. Coyne (1989) concluded that 'studies that have attempted to identify a persistent traitlike quality to depressive cognitions have generated considerable evidence to the contrary'.

Obsessions That Are Not Doubted

Views on obsessions have been remarkably consistent over a long period of time. Current definitions, such as those in DSM-5, the *International Classification of Diseases, Tenth Edition* (ICD-10) and any number of textbooks of psychiatry, identify them as ideas, thoughts, impulses or images which are recurrent and intrusive, and which the individual considers senseless and tries to ignore or suppress. This definition can be traced back to Schneider (1930) who described obsessions as 'contents of consciousness which, when they occur, are accompanied by the experience of subjective compulsion, and which cannot be got rid of, though on quiet reflection they are recognized as senseless'; and then further to Esquirol in the nineteenth century who considered them to be ideas, images, feelings or movements accompanied by a sense of compulsion and a desire to resist them, with the individual recognizing them as foreign to his personality.

In the way of textbook definitions, however, the idea that patients with obsessive-compulsive disorder do not believe that their obsessions are really true is an oversimplification.

This was first pointed out by Lewis (the same Lewis who carried out the aforesaid study of melancholia) in what remains one of the most eloquent and insightful analyses of the phenomenology of obsessions. For him (Lewis, 1957), the important feature was the patient's struggle against the thought:

> The indispensable subjective component of an obsession lies in the consciousness of the patient: to him it is an act of will, which he cannot help making, to try and suppress or destroy the unwelcome intruder upon his mental integrity; but the effort is always in vain. It does not matter whether the intruder is a thought, an idea, or an image, or an impulse, accompanied by appropriate affect. Along with this subjective feeling of compulsion goes an inability to accept the experience as part of one's proper and integrated mental activity: it is a foreign body, not implanted from without (as a disordered schizophrenic experience might be held to be by the patient) but arising from within, homemade but disowned, a sort of mental sequestrum, a calculus that keeps on causing trouble.

In contrast, he (Lewis, 1936) considered recognition of the senselessness of the idea to be non-essential:

> Critical appraisal of the obsession, and recognition that it is absurd represents a defensive, intellectual effort, intended to destroy it: it is not always present, nor is the obsessional idea always absurd.

Here, Lewis was ahead of his time: starting approximately 50 years later there has been a steady stream of publications reporting that some patients with otherwise typical obsessive-compulsive disorder do not consider their obsessions to be unreasonable. This phenomenon is most commonly referred to as lack of insight into obsessions, but also as development of overvalued ideation (Kozak & Foa, 1994), or as obsessive-compulsive disorder with psychotic features (Solyom et al., 1985; Insel & Akiskal, 1986; Eisen & Rasmussen, 1993). At a rough guess, it is probably seen in around 10 per cent of patients with the disorder, although the variation around this figure was wide in three large surveys (Eisen & Rasmussen, 1993; Foa et al., 1995; Catapano et al., 2001). This uncertainty almost certainly reflects what the authors of these surveys were prepared to accept as evidence of the obsession not being considered irrational, from patients actually believing that the feared consequence would actually occur if a ritual was not performed, to feeling that the obsession was reasonable, to defending their beliefs against counterargument.

It has to be said that not all the examples of this phenomenon that have been described are convincing. Thus, in one of the seminal articles on the subject, Insel and Akiskal (1986) described four patients. One of them recognized that his obsession about contamination with germs was irrational, but he was considered to show a commitment to it by virtue of the fact that he covertly wore surgical gloves and stuffed his sheets into the hospital incinerator every morning – hardly unusual behaviour in obsessive-compulsive disorder. In another influential account Solyom et al. (1985) described a group of eight patients who had obsessions with no feeling of subjective compulsion and without insight and resistance. However, three were described as having disturbance of body image as their major symptom, raising the possibility that they might have been better diagnosed as suffering from body dysmorphic disorder. Another of the patients was described as having a hypochondriacal obsession; here it seems possible that the diagnosis could have been hypochondriasis: patients with this latter diagnosis are often misdiagnosed as having obsessive-compulsive disorder before the clinician belatedly realizes his or her mistake (the present author has done this several times). Nevertheless, there is no doubt that patients exist who truly believe that their obsessions are rational. An example is shown in Box 2.4.

Box 2.4 A Patient Who Firmly Believed in Her Obsessions (Reproduced with permission from Foa, 1979)

Judy was a 37-year-old artist, married to a businessman. They had three children, ages eight, six and three. She was afraid of being contaminated by leukaemia germs which she would then transmit to her children and husband. She described the following at her first interview with her therapist:

T. I understand that you need to wash excessively everytime you are in contact, direct or indirect, with leukemia.

P. Yes, like the other day I was sitting in the beauty parlor, and I heard the woman who sat next to me telling this other woman that she had just come back from the Children's Hospital where she had visited her grandson who had leukemia. I immediately left, I registered in a hotel, and washed for three days.

T. What do you think would have happened if you did not wash?

P. My children and my husband would get leukemia and die.

T. Would you die too?

P. No, because I am immune, but they are particularly susceptible to these germs.

T. Do you really think people get leukemia through germs?

P. I have talked with several specialists about it. They all tried to assure me that there are no leukemia germs, but medicine is not that advanced; I am convinced that I know something that the doctors have not yet discovered. There are definitely germs that carry leukemia.

T. What is the probability that if you didn't wash after the incident in the beauty parlor your family would get leukemia?

P. One hundred per cent. They might not get it immediately, these germs could be in their bodies for five or even ten years. Eventually they will have leukaemia. So you see, if I don't wash, it's as if I murdered them.

In a few cases the ideas enter very strange territory indeed. O'Dwyer and Marks (2000) described a series of five patients who had elaborate beliefs in the context of what were otherwise clear-cut obsessive-compulsive illnesses. One of these was a young man with rituals which completely dominated his life. These related to a 'power' he believed he had, which he felt brought him luck and he was in constant danger of losing. He also believed there was a second power of evil, possessed by a workman, and he developed a separate set of rituals to ward this off. He believed implicitly in these powers and feared terrible consequences for him and his family if he did not retain the former and repel the latter. On one occasion, at the beginning of his illness he had seen a man's face at a glass door and heard a voice say, 'Do the habits and things will go right.' He also claimed that when he experienced loss of the good power, he would see a black dot about the size of his fist leaving his body. Another patient, a man in his late thirties, had the fear that reflections in mirrors represented another world and developed rituals in relation to this. He feared being transported into this other world and sometimes believed that he had actually been transported there: when this happened he believed he would be forced to stay there if he ate while in it. The other world looked the same as the real one, but 'felt' different and he wondered whether his family and friends had been replaced by identical appearing doubles. Both patients failed to respond to antipsychotic drug treatment, but the first improved markedly on treatment with clomipramine and behaviour therapy, and the second improved moderately on behaviour therapy alone.

All this naturally raises the question of whether there is some kind of deep link between obsessions and delusions. This view gains strength from claims, made from the nineteenth century onwards, that obsessions can sometimes transform into delusions (see Rosen, 1957;

Burgy, 2007). This is said to happen when a patient with obsessive-compulsive disorder develops major depression, or when an illness that starts off as obsessional later reveals itself to be schizophrenia, both of which are well-documented occurrences (e.g. Stengel, 1945; Gittleson, 1966). Bleuler (1924) was an early supporter of this view. On the other hand, Schneider (1925, quoted by Burgy, 2007), denied that such transitions ever occurred.

Gordon (1926) set out to answer the question empirically. He collected a series of six patients with obsessive-compulsive disorder who later developed delusions, in most cases in the context of a depressive illness. He found a reasonably direct relationship between the content of the obsession and the content of the delusion in one case. This was a 13-year-old girl who developed obsessional doubts about whether she had carried out actions like writing, speaking and walking correctly, and would have to repeat the actions several times before she was satisfied. At the age of 18 she started working as a kindergarten teacher, and shortly afterwards began to dwell on the idea that she was not teaching her pupils correctly. This then became a conviction that she had taught her pupils the opposite of what they needed to know, and that she would be dismissed and would never be able to work again. She later started to hear the children's voices reproaching her and then God's voice telling her that both she and her parents would be sacrificed.

In two other patients the link was less straightforward. One had longstanding hypochondriacal preoccupations about the function of his intestines, liver and kidneys, 'which he genuinely doubted'. Several years later he developed persecutory and referential delusions, probably in the context of major depression, and came to believe that he was correct about his previous health concerns. The other patient had experienced a compulsion to repeat his prayers without missing out a word for two years. Towards the end of this period he gradually developed an explanation for doing this, that since he had to pray there must be some divine reason for it. He went on to believe he was a sinner and deserved everything that happened to him or would happen to him. He no longer questioned the necessity of praying. He later developed visual and auditory hallucinations.

Further studies are decidedly thin on the ground. Those that the present author has been able to find are summarized in Table 2.2. In most cases the link is less than direct or there is some other complication. Thus, one of Stengel's (1945) patients had had sadistic and blasphemous thoughts from childhood which included violent ideas towards women. In adult life he developed a paranoid illness where one of his beliefs was that women were the cause of all the evil in the world. Stengel (1945) considered that the delusion was not a derivative of the obsession, although the contents of both were related to the patient's underlying impulses and complexes. In another of his cases, a woman started washing her hands compulsively in response to a fear of germs and also of dog excrement and earthworms. Seven years later she developed an illness that was probably schizophrenia. One of her symptoms was eating dead flies, earthworms and animal excrement, which she explained was to glorify God by humiliating herself and doing things she abhorred.

Rosen (1957) described four apparent transitions in an examination of the case notes of 30 schizophrenic patients who had at some point experienced obsessions. In two, it was clearly not a case of direct transformation. One patient had fears of contamination and harm through loose objects lying about and later developed beliefs about being poisoned and had hallucinations of people falling off roofs and being pushed down drains. The other, a woman who initially had a compulsive urge to look at men's genitals later came to believe that everyone knew that she had this compulsion. In a third patient, the transition was not to delusions: a patient who had previously experienced single words coming into her mind later developed thought

Table 2.2 Studies of Obsessions That Convert to Delusions

Study	Patients	Direct Link between Obsession and Delusion	Indirect Link between Obsession and Delusion	Comment
Gordon (1926)	Six obsessive-compulsive patients who developed major depression or schizophrenia	1	2	See text
Stengel (1945)	Fourteen patients in whom obsessional symptoms preceded depression or schizophrenia	0	2	See text
Rosen (1957)	Thirty schizophrenic patients in whom obsessional symptoms had been observed at some point	?1 (not clear if the patient had actually developed schizophrenia)	2	See text
Goldberg (1965)	Four patients with mixed obsessional and paranoid symptoms over many years	0	0	Three cases were of morbid jealousy; the fourth simply had an obsessional fear that he was suspected of theft.
Robinson et al. (1976)	Three cases of 'obsessive psychosis'	0	0	The patients all lacked insight into their obsessions, leading to a diagnosis of psychosis being made on psychoanalytic grounds.
Insel and Akiskal (1986)	Four cases of obsessive compulsive disorder with psychotic features	1	0	See text

insertion which sometimes included the same words. The most direct link was in a patient who developed an obsession that she might harm someone and four years later started to believe that she might harm God; she also began hearing His voice saying this. However, it is not altogether certain that this patient had actually developed schizophrenia: although she expressed the belief that she might harm God, she carried on performing rituals in response to this idea and was aware of the absurdity of it. The author's statement that the patient 'was not entirely convinced that the hallucinations were due to her imagination' might also raise doubts about whether what she was experiencing was truly hallucinatory in nature.

In Insel and Akiskal's (1986) series of four patients, a link between the content of the obsession and the content of the delusion was considered to be present in only one. This was a patient with a long history of obsessive checking who became preoccupied with the idea that he may have inadvertently poisoned the children's juice in the day centre where he worked. Later he was admitted and while in hospital developed a short-lived psychotic state. As part of this, he became convinced that the hospital staff in collusion the FBI believed he had committed this crime. However, he maintained that he did not do this.

Conclusion: The Complexity of Pathological Belief

The simple answer to the question of when a delusion is not a delusion is 'When it is an overvalued idea'. Despite being ignored, misunderstood and lost altogether on American psychiatry (it is difficult to resist the temptation to say undervalued), there seems to be a clear need for such a second category of abnormal belief. Trying to deny its existence simply leads to contradictions, of which the nature of the belief in anorexia nervosa is the most glaring example. In an ideal world, it might be better to start afresh with a different name for this form of psychopathology, such as quasi-delusions, or non-psychotic delusions, or even perhaps type II abnormal beliefs. But the fact is that the term overvalued idea not only has the force of history behind it, but also actually captures the phenomenological features of the symptom quite nicely.

Whatever else it is, the overvalued idea is not a halfway house between normal beliefs and delusions. However, a form of abnormal belief that gives an almost irresistible impression of being so exists in the ideas of hopelessness, self-depreciation and self-blame seen in major depression – Beck's depressive cognitions – and the corresponding grandiose ideas in mania. Does this mean that all delusions, not just those seen in major affective disorder, are on a continuum with other less pathological ideas, perhaps even with beliefs we all hold at certain times? This seems on the face of it to go against the conclusions reached about the nature of delusions in Chapter 1. On the other hand it is the position taken by a currently highly influential theory, the so-called continuum view of psychosis, which is considered in detail in Chapter 4.

If there are some types of abnormal belief that are not on a continuum with delusions and some that are, where do obsessions stand? On balance, the evidence seems to be more in line the former. There can be no doubt that obsessions are sometimes held with firm conviction. However, in most cases where this happens the beliefs continue to look like obsessions rather than, say, overvalued ideas – the patient in Box 2.4, for example, still responded to her idea about 'leukaemia germs' by performing compulsive rituals and did not develop a hypochondriasis-like pattern of help-seeking behaviour. Rarely, as in the cases described by O'Dwyer and Marks (2000), the beliefs go further, to the point that the patient seems to be fully committed to what might be termed an obsessional fantasy world. But even here the resulting state does not seem to resemble psychosis in key ways, not least its response to treatment. The acid test of the existence of a continuum between obsessions and delusions is whether the former can sometimes transform into the latter. Given that only at most two or three convincing examples of this phenomenon have ever been recorded, the verdict here has to be one of 'not proven'.

Delusional Disorder

So far the contours of abnormal belief seem reasonably well defined. On the one hand there are delusions, as seen in schizophrenia and psychotic forms of mania and depression. On the other hand there is a miscellany of other forms of abnormal belief, the most important of which is the overvalued idea. However, a further psychiatric presentation, paranoia or delusional disorder as it is now known, has the potential to undermine this simple scheme. As well as presenting an enduring challenge from the nosological point of view, there are real questions about whether patients with the disorder are deluded in quite the same way as those with, say, schizophrenia. Nor is it clear whether the various subtypes of delusional disorder are consistent with each other in this respect. Finally, the question of whether delusions are just one end of a spectrum of abnormal belief, touched on in Chapter 2, raises its head again here.

As with just about everything else in psychiatry, the modern history of delusional disorder began with Kraepelin. After giving the first descriptions of the disorders now known as schizophrenia and bipolar disorder, he turned his attention to a diagnostic concept that was already in existence, paranoia. This, he noted (Kraepelin, 1913b), was supposed to refer to patients who showed a well-organized set of delusions in the absence of other symptoms; however, over the preceding century use of the term had become so debased that it was being applied to 70–80 per cent of patients in German mental hospitals, many of whom showed 'only a few, meagre, disconnected or confused delusions'. Nevertheless, by 1913 he (Kraepelin, 1913b) had managed to identify a small number of patients – 19 according to a later follow-up study by Kolle (1931) – with the requisite clinical features. They all showed insidiously developing well-formed delusions; hallucinations were at most minor, and on matters unrelated to their delusions the patients remained completely rational.

It was clear from the outset, however, that the borders of paranoia were not going to be easy to defend. One obvious question concerned its distinction from schizophrenia. Kraepelin (1913b) felt that progression to this disorder did not occur: among other things he pointed to the case of a woman who had become ill at the age of 45 and who he had had the opportunity to observe until she was in her nineties. She remained deluded but otherwise, apart from a certain senile forgetfulness, there was no sign of even mild schizophrenia-like symptomatology. Bleuler (1911), however, was not sure that the possibility could be ruled out that paranoia was simply a form of schizophrenia that was so mild that it could just about lead to delusional ideas. This latter view gradually gained the upper hand, to the extent that by 1958 Schneider (quoted by Marneros et al., 2012) was able to state confidently: 'Paranoia is dead. It is simply schizophrenia.'

Another area of contention was the kind of presentation exemplified by the querulous paranoid state. As described in Chapter 2, Kraepelin (1913b) ultimately felt it necessary to exclude such patients from the category of paranoia on the grounds that their illnesses seemed clearly to be a response to external factors rather than the result of some internal pathological process. In doing so, he opened the door for a later author, Kretschmer (1927) to argue that individuals with certain 'sensitive' personality traits (shyness, insecurity and a tendency to feel emotions deeply to the point of being consumed by them) could develop delusions when faced with conflicts they could not cope with. These were not delusions in quite the same way as those seen in schizophrenia, however, and the patient could make a full recovery from them. His views went on to become influential in British and European psychiatry.

By the mid-1970s, paranoia had lapsed back into the same terminological inexactitude that had characterized much of its earlier history. The leading international disease classification of the day, ICD-9, listed three categories of paranoid illness: paranoia, considered to be rare, a paranoid 'state' in which delusions were the main but not necessarily the only symptom, and paraphrenia (see Chapter 1). The features that distinguished these states from each other were not at all clearly articulated, particularly with respect to the question of whether or not patients were allowed to have hallucinations. British views of the day were represented by Forrest (1975, 1978), one of the editors of a well-regarded textbook of psychiatry: what he called paranoid psychosis was an illness that developed after the age of 30 in which there were persecutory or other delusions and auditory hallucinations; there could even be Schneiderian first rank symptoms in some cases. In some patients, particularly women in their forties, there was also a clear depressive element to the illness. Consulting the relevant American literature on paranoia during this period was not advisable.

Nevertheless, it was in America, or at any rate the North American continent, where a series of events took place that would lead to paranoia re-establishing itself as a credible diagnosis. Winokur (1977) reviewed the case notes of patients in the large mental hospital where he worked and was able to find 29 patients who conformed closely to Kraepelin's (1913b) description of the disorder. Around the same time a Canadian psychiatrist Munro and his co-workers (Riding & Munro, 1975a,b; Munro, 1978) started to publish on a disorder that seemed to show the features of a hypochondriacal form of paranoia, something that Kraepelin (1913b) felt existed, but which he had not actually seen. Ultimately, another American psychiatrist, Kendler (1980), reviewed a number of studies of paranoia that had been carried out over the years and, almost certainly also influenced by the work of Munro, decided that there was enough evidence to propose a provisional set of diagnostic criteria for what he decided to call simple delusional disorder. With its name shortened slightly to delusional disorder, this was then officially incorporated into the first revision of DSM-III, DSM-III-R in 1987.

None of which should be taken to mean that the nosological uncertainties associated with paranoia have gone away. The longstanding question of whether and to what extent delusional disorder is separate from schizophrenia remains, despite new research, not fully resolved. The existence of an association with affective disorder, an issue that was first mooted in the British literature, now looms large, with statements to this effect being present in both the DSM-5 and ICD-10 criteria for the disorder. Perhaps most importantly, from DSM-III-R onwards, American psychiatry has been steadily tying itself in knots over what to do when patients with body dysmorphic disorder appear completely convinced that their beliefs are true and so on the face of it warrant a diagnosis of delusional disorder. Dealing with these issues is not easy, and the only way to get to the bottom of them is to retrace the key historical steps that have taken place from Kraepelin (1913b) onwards.

Kraepelinian Paranoia

For Kraepelin (1913b), the essential feature of paranoia was the insidious development of delusions in the absence of other psychotic symptoms or other features suggestive of a diagnosis of schizophrenia. Auditory hallucinations, in particular, only occurred in exceptional circumstances, perhaps in a dream-like state or as a visionary experience in the early stages of the disorder – one of the examples he gave was of a patient with future religious delusions whose illness began when he saw Christ and at the same time heard a voice saying 'Feed my sheep.' Nor did the patients show evidence of the flattening or inappropriateness of affect typically seen in schizophrenia. Their behaviour could certainly be influenced by their beliefs, so that they regularly did things like placing adverts in newspapers, complaining to the police or attempting to force entry into the premises of highly placed persons. However, on matters not touching on their delusions there was a 'perfect preservation of clear and orderly thinking, willing, and acting'.

The delusions themselves were systematized; that is, they were logical, well integrated and without gross internal contradictions:

> The patients exert themselves to gain a picture, certainly distorted in an extremely ego-centric fashion, of their place in the mechanism of life, a kind of view of the universe. They bring their experiences into relation with each other, they search for cause and effect, for motives and connections. Obscure points and contradictions are as far as possible set aside and smoothed over by laborious thought, so that a delusional structure arises, which, however, with all the improbability and uncertainty of its foundations, does not usually contain any apparent absolute impossibilities.

For Kraepelin (1913b), there were two fundamental directions the delusions could take, persecutory and expansive or grandiose. The persecutory form, which appeared to be the most frequent type, typically began with delusions of reference and misinterpretation. The patients would start to notice that people no longer seemed as friendly as previously. This would then progress to feelings that they were being laughed at behind their back and that remarks were being passed about them. Letters directed to them would be opened and stolen. If they changed their place of residence, they would soon begin to notice that people seemed to have complete information about them.

Eventually an explanation of all that was happening would become clear. This could occur suddenly ('scales seem to fall from their eyes, secret connections become clear to them like lightning'), but more typically the realization dawned slowly, sometimes taking years. Thereafter, both the central delusion and the delusions of reference and misinterpretation that gave rise to it would continue in a mutually reinforcing web of belief.

In the jealous form, the patient – a man in most of Kraepelin's (1913b) cases – would start to notice all kinds of occurrences that gradually strengthened his belief that his wife was being unfaithful to him. She might seem cold, or reject his advances, or she would start going out for long periods at unusual hours; suspicious men would come to the house asking for her on various pretexts and he would notice people alluding to her infidelity in what they said. The accusations of unfaithfulness that followed were often extravagant: she had multiple lovers, was having sex with hawkers and lodgers, or was even committing incest with her sons. Sometimes the delusions would be near-impossible – one patient claimed he saw his brother having sex with his wife through the sitting room door, and another described how his wife would place a cloth over his face in bed prior to consorting with her lover.

An introductory phase of delusions of reference and misinterpretation was also characteristic of the group of patients with delusions of high descent. The idea often first arose when they heard their parents whispering in an adjoining room or started greeting them with peculiar seriousness, or when they saw a surprising resemblance to themselves in a bust or a portrait. Thereafter, they would notice occurrences such as strangers taking off their hats to them or the band in the theatre beginning to play as soon they appeared. When the patients tried to assert their birthright, they would encounter all kinds of subtle interventions from the aristocratic family concerned designed to prevent them from doing so. Sometimes the interventions were not so subtle, when, as often happened, they found themselves committed to an asylum. Delusional memories could also be prominent in this form of paranoia: one patient remembered how as a small child he lived in a beautiful castle before being taken away and could describe the magnificent furniture and decoration of the rooms.

In contrast, referentiality was considerably less pronounced in two other forms of paranoia. The religious form sometimes began with the kind of isolated visionary experiences noted previously – one patient saw the sun rising like an egg and noticed that a gloriole surrounded him, and another experienced or perhaps remembered an event where he was levitated off the ground in church. The patients' subsequent religious convictions could at first be difficult to distinguish from genuine religious awakenings, and not infrequently they attracted groups of followers. But the delusional nature of the belief sooner or later revealed itself when, for example, the patients started maintaining that they could prophesize events such as earthquakes or that they did not need to read newspapers to know what is going on in the world. One patient found that if he said something beautiful, he would meet a beautiful man with a lilac-coloured tie, otherwise it would be an ugly man with an unpleasant one. Another patient attributed secret significance to the colour and appearance of the dogs he saw the street.

The group of deluded or cranky inventors were perhaps the most difficult to diagnose. Although their ideas often took the form of perpetual motion machines and the like, sometimes the devices were quite mundane and practicable – Kraepelin (1913b) mentioned a boot with a jointed sole, an electrical regulator of beer pressure and a condenser for a refrigerator. A more reliable guide to their pathological nature was the patients' unshakeable belief in the large amounts of money they were going to make from the invention. This would lead them to do things like demand support from the state or make marriage proposals to women they had never met. As in the religious form, delusions of reference and misinterpretation tended to enter the picture late, especially when the patients started to see what they considered to be the results of their ideas stolen by others and already in use.

Lastly, Kraepelin (1913b) described a delusional form of erotomania. Here, in contrast to the form of the disorder described in Chapter 2, the patient would see evidence of the other person's romantic interest wherever he or she (at least as many of Kraepelin's cases were male as female) went, and would receive information about the other's intentions in a roundabout way:

> His love is an open secret and an object of universal interest; it is talked about everywhere, certainly never outspokenly but always only in slight indications, the profound meaning of which he understands very well ... Of course, this extraordinary love must meantime be kept secret; therefore, the patient receives all messages in indirect ways, always through the mediation of others, by the newspapers, and in the form of concealed remarks.

Importantly in view of later developments, Kraepelin (1913b) was also in favour of a hypochondriacal form of paranoia existing. He had not personally seen a case characterized only or predominantly by this type of delusion, but such beliefs were certainly present in the background in the other types, with patients often complaining that their memory was failing or that they had pains in various parts of his body which meant that they were seriously ill. Indeed none of the different varieties of paranoia were sharply demarcated from each other: patients with the persecutory form frequently also developed exaggerated ideas of their own abilities and occasionally had co-existing delusions of jealousy. Cranky inventors would come to feel that they had been duped out of their rewards by hostile machinations. In erotomania love could turn to hate and lead to a delusion of persecution.

According to Kraepelin (1913b), the delusions of patients with paranoia typically remained unchanged for years or decades. Ultimately, the central belief might become more indistinct and nonsensical, and lose its influence over behaviour; however, weakmindedness – Kraepelin's term for the milder forms of deterioration in schizophrenia – or other psychotic symptoms never seemed to develop.

Whether this was truly the case was examined some years later by Kolle (1931), who reviewed the case notes of 19 patients diagnosed as suffering from paranoia by Kraepelin and his colleagues, 4 to 22 years after the diagnosis was originally made. He found that one patient later became prone to talking incoherently about Hitler and other topics. Another developed a bizarre belief that he was being affected by radiation and had felt blows to his chest. Yet another became withdrawn and lived a hermit-like existence. In another 10 cases no major changes in the clinical picture took place. Here, though, Kolle (1931) mounted a convoluted argument roughly to the effect that these patients' delusions actually showed, or came to show, the kind of internal contradictions and impossibilities typical of delusions in schizophrenia. The remaining patients were excluded by Kolle (1931) from his analysis for various reasons; interestingly, in two cases this was because Kraepelin had added the qualification of 'manic predisposition' or 'possible manic-depressive psychosis' to their diagnoses.

Kraepelin (1913b) himself pointed out another problem for the concept of paranoia, the fact that patients existed who showed the rudiments of paranoia without developing actual delusions. In addition to the obvious example of the querulous paranoid state, he also noted individuals who developed ideas rather than frank delusions about their partners being unfaithful. Others determinedly pursued unlikely inventions and money-making schemes, or worked on lofty plans to benefit mankind, which were out of proportion to their knowledge and ability. He had also seen patients who, in a way reminiscent of erotomania, relentlessly pursued a person of the opposite sex, in spite of the most unequivocal refusals. In all these cases, the beliefs were somehow vaguer and more indefinite than in paranoia; they appeared and receded again without disappearing altogether; and they 'consisted in a strong personal valuation of actual events, which was not too far removed from the one-sidedness of normal individuals'. Unlike the question of paranoia's separation from schizophrenia, this issue would remain dormant for many years.

Munro's Monosymptomatic Hypochondriacal Psychosis

As paranoia lapsed back into nosological confusion in the decades following Kraepelin's (1913b) description, there was very little in the way of new findings or rigorous debate. Change, when it did come, was from an unexpected direction. In 1971, Munro saw his first case of what appeared to be an example of the hypochondriacal form of paranoia alluded to by Kraepelin. At the time he was not aware that such a disorder existed, something he considered to be due to the English language literature having all but suppressed Kraepelin's thinking on the subject. He went on to describe his experience with increasing numbers of cases of what he called monosymptomatic hypochondriacal psychosis in a series of papers (Riding and Munro, 1975a,b; Munro, 1978, 1980,1988; Munro and Chmara, 1982), a monograph (Munro, 1982) and finally a book (Munro, 1999).

In the first of these papers (Riding & Munro, 1975), he and a colleague reported four cases. The first was a 42-year-old man who had started to believe that he gave off an unpleasant smell. The second was a 20-year-old man who was convinced that people were looking at his neck and who had previously had similar concerns about his nose. The third was a 57-year-old man who believed he was infested with bugs, which he could feel moving under his skin. The fourth was similar to the second in that he believed he had intermittent facial swelling which made him ugly. These four cases are summarized in Box 3.1. There was also a fifth case, an elderly woman who complained about tiny beasts crawling out of her umbilicus, but there were some doubts about her diagnosis as she showed evidence of peripheral arteriosclerosis, although her orientation and her memory were not impaired.

Box 3.1 Munro's First Four Cases of Monosymptomatic Hypochondriacal Psychosis (Reproduced with Permission from Riding & Munro, 1975a)

Case 1

Over a six-month period a 42-year-old single man started to believe that he gave off an unpleasant smell. He complained increasingly about the smell, which he believed was due to flatus and had recently stopped mixing with friends and workmates. He had previously been a heavy drinker, and had suffered a head injury resulting in brief unconsciousness, but there was no other psychiatric history. There was no evidence of depression on examination and no other symptoms. Treatment with three different antipsychotic drugs was tried but caused excessive tiredness. He was put on a low dose of a further antipsychotic drug, pimozide, and within a few days the delusion had disappeared. The patient returned to work, mixed freely in company and reported that he was more self-assertive than previously. The belief returned five months later when he stopped taking treatment but promptly disappeared again when he resumed taking it. He remained well for two years but suffered two depressive episodes, which required treatment with antidepressants.

Case 2

A 20-year-old single man developed the belief in adolescence that people looked at him and talked about him because of the shape of his nose. At the age of 18 he underwent cosmetic surgery for this. Thereafter, he became convinced that people were now looking at his neck, which he felt was abnormally long. He began to wear very high collars and gave up work. His neck was physically normal but he could not be convinced of this. There was no other abnormality apart from this single unshakeable belief on examination, although he showed an indefinable oddness of manner. After three weeks on pimozide, the patient was markedly improved: tension was less and he was less worried about people looking at him. Four months after beginning treatment he agreed that his neck was normal and that he had possibly been overconcerned about his nose in the past. He had obtained a new job and was planning to expand his social life.

Case 3

A 57-year-old man had been well until 18 months previously, when he started to believe his head was infested with insects. He washed and shaved his head repeatedly and could feel the insects moving under his skin. He had isolated himself from his family, fearful of contaminating them. He brought an envelope to the clinic containing skin flakes, which he said were eggs. He had been a very heavy drinker when younger but in recent years drank moderately. He had a medical history of protein-losing enteropathy and had been taking steroids for four years. He showed a degree of anxiety over the delusion about parasites, but there was no evidence of depressive illness or any other psychiatric abnormality. After around four months of treatment, complicated by a period of non-compliance, he was increasingly convinced that he was parasite-free and no longer spent time washing excessively and shaving his head.

Case 4

A 20-year-old unmarried man complained of intermittent facial swelling which made him ugly. The symptom had begun a year earlier following a car accident in which he had been unconscious for 30 minutes. He kept his hair brushed over his face and had strong ideas of reference. He was noted to be depressed on examination, but after 5 weeks of treatment on a tricyclic antidepressant, he was even more deluded. The diagnosis of depression was therefore revised and he was started on pimozide. Within a week the patient was more cheerful, had begun to show his face and go out, and seemed to be gaining insight regarding his appearance. Two weeks later he was working and leading a normal social life, was no longer depressed and only rarely thought of his appearance.

Riding and Munro (1975) argued that these patients had in common a hypochondriacal complaint which they were utterly convinced about, but which could not be attributed to another diagnosis such as schizophrenia or major depression. That the belief was essentially delusional in nature was further reinforced by the fact that they all showed a prompt and excellent response to treatment with an antipsychotic drug, pimozide.

Munro was well aware that one or two issues remained to be clarified. One of these concerned the possible alternative diagnosis of depression. Riding and Munro's (1975) fourth case was significantly depressed at the time of presentation, and a provisional diagnosis of major depression had even been made. However, they were sceptical that this diagnosis was correct, because the patient became worse when treated with an antidepressant but then responded dramatically to pimozide. Another patient (Case 1) experienced two episodes of depression after he had improved on treatment with pimozide, which both responded to treatment with antidepressants. Riding and Munro (1975) were inclined to think that the depression in this case was a side effect of antipsychotic treatment.

Later, in his monograph describing 50 cases, Munro (1982) noted that six patients developed depression at some point during their recovery, and that some had also shown a slight lessening of their delusional preoccupation while on antidepressant treatment alone. Case reports by other authors also described more substantial improvement with antidepressant treatment in patients with monsymptomatic hypochondriacal psychosis (Roberts & Roberts, 1977; Cashman & Pollock, 1983). These considerations ultimately led Munro (1999) to the conclusion that '[delusional] and mood disorders are separate illnesses with their own natural histories and treatment responses, but there is a relationship, albeit a subtle and complex one, between them'.

The other issue requiring attention was why Cases 2 and 4 could not simply have been suffering from body dysmorphic disorder. Riding and Munro (1975) countered that the literature at the time (e.g. Hay, 1970; Andreasen & Bardach, 1977) clearly encompassed both psychotic ('dysmorphic delusion') and non-psychotic ('dysmorphic neurosis') forms of these disorders. Similar heterogeneity was also evident in cases of the infestation syndrome (Skott, 1978). Twenty years later, the line Munro took on this issue would come back to haunt him.

Winokur and Kendler: Delusional Disorder

While Munro was arguing for the existence of monosymptomatic hypochondriacal psychosis, across the border in America revolution was in the air. A group of psychiatrists who believed in a scientific psychiatry founded on descriptive principles was plotting to overthrow the dominant psychoanalytic establishment, which in recent years had led to the country becoming the psychiatric equivalent of a pariah state. One of the members of what was later to be called the neo-Kraepelinian movement (Blashfield, 1984) was Winokur. In 1977 he published the results of a study where he examined the case records of the Psychiatric Hospital of the University of Iowa, which had a reputation for being very detailed, and found 29 patients who seemed to correspond to paranoia as described by Kraepelin (1913b). They mostly showed persecutory, jealous and referential delusions, but there were a few with grandiose or hypochondriacal forms of illness. Follow-up of 26 of these patients for an average of 2.6 years (and much longer in some cases) revealed that on the whole the diagnosis did not change, although one patient became obviously schizophrenic and another was subsequently given a diagnosis of manic-depressive psychosis, depressed type (a term in use at the time for major depression). Winokur (1977) suggested the term delusional disorder for this presentation, partly to avoid restricting the concept of the disorder just to states where there were persecutory delusions.

Three years later, a palace coup had taken place in the headquarters of the American Psychiatric Association (graphically described by Wilson, 1993), and American psychiatry was in the hands of the neo-Kraepelinians. All diagnoses now had to be made on the basis of the presenting clinical symptoms, not hypothetical underlying psychological mechanisms that the clinician intuited to be present. To assist with this there was a new and much expanded third edition of the American Diagnostic and Statistical Manual, the landmark DSM-III. Paranoia was included as a subcategory of paranoid disorders, where it resembled the illness described by Kraepelin: there had to be a stable delusional system of at least six months' duration in the absence of schizophrenic symptoms or a full depressive or manic syndrome. However, the diagnostic criteria only allowed persecutory or jealous delusions.

The same year that DSM-III appeared, another phenomenologically minded American psychiatrist, Kendler (1980), reviewed existing studies where the definition of paranoia conformed reasonably well to a set of criteria similar to those used by Winokur (1977). The central requirement was presence of delusions of any type (i.e. not just persecutory) and/or persistent pervasive ideas of reference, in the absence of hallucinations or other symptoms suggestive of schizophrenia such as formal thought disorder and first-rank symptoms. It was also stipulated that the delusions should be 'non-bizarre' (bizarre or multiple delusions were a criterion for schizophrenia in DSM-III). Finally, there should be no evidence of acute or chronic organic brain disease, and a full affective syndrome, either depressive or manic, had to be absent at the time the patient was delusional.

Kendler was able to find 17 studies that fulfilled most or all of these criteria; the earliest was Kolle's (1931) follow-up of Kraepelin's patients and the most recent was that of Winokur (1977); Riding and Munro's (1975) study was also included. Across the studies the peak age of onset was in the late thirties to mid-forties and 60 per cent to 80 per cent of patients were married; this was a demographic signature quite different from that of schizophrenia. After their index admission approximately a third of patients had no further hospitalizations, and two-thirds remained employed much of the time, something that again would be highly unusual for schizophrenia. On follow-up, a large majority of patients retained the same diagnosis over periods ranging from a few months to 20 years. With regard to family history, the evidence was limited and inconclusive: two out of three studies found an elevated rate of schizophrenia in first degree relatives, and none of them found an increased risk of affective disorder. Overall, Kendler (1980) concluded that it was both plausible and parsimonious to consider delusional disorder as a disorder in its own right.

When DSM-III-R appeared seven years later, the section for paranoid disorders had been scrapped and delusional disorder now had its own category. Grandiose and hypochondriacal delusions were permitted, the latter as delusional disorder somatic type. Co-existent major affective disorder was not an exclusion criterion, although such episodes were required to be brief in comparison to the period of delusional symptoms. The criteria were not changed in DSM-IV when it came out in 1994, and ICD-10, which was also introduced in the 1990s, followed them closely.

The current DSM-5 criteria for delusional disorder are not very different and are shown in Box 3.2. The main change is that the requirement for the delusions to be non-bizarre has been removed and replaced by a 'specifier' to be added when this is not the case. Also worthy of note is the statement that the symptoms are not better explained by another disorder, such as body dysmorphic disorder or obsessive-compulsive disorder.

Box 3.2 DSM-5 Criteria for Delusional Disorder

A. The presence of one (or more) delusions with a duration of 1 month or longer.

B. Criterion A for schizophrenia has never been met.

Note: Hallucinations, if present, are not prominent and are related to the delusional theme (e.g., the sensation of being infested with insects associated with delusions of infestation).

C. Apart from the impact of the delusion(s) or its ramifications, functioning is not markedly impaired, and behavior is not obviously bizarre or odd.

D. If manic or major depressive episodes have occurred, these have been brief relative to the duration of the delusional periods.

E. The disturbance is not attributable to the physiological effects of a substance or another medical condition and is not better explained by another mental disorder, such as body dysmorphic disorder or obsessive-compulsive disorder.

Beyond DSM-5: The Problems Facing Delusional Disorder

One issue that Kendler did not feel had been satisfactorily answered in his 1980 review was whether delusional disorder was really a mild form of schizophrenia which ran a benign clinical course. Although the four studies that included follow-up data all found that a large majority of the patients retained their initial diagnosis, all of them also found that some patients ultimately developed schizophrenia – 3 per cent, 12 per cent, 13 per cent and 22 per cent respectively. The studies themselves were not without weaknesses: one only contained nine patients and in the others the follow-up period was relatively short for at least some of the patients.

Since then, something approximating to a definitive study has been carried out. The Halle Delusional Syndromes (HADES) study (Marneros et al., 2012; see also Marneros, 2012; Wustmann et al., 2012) screened for patients with delusional disorder by reviewing the case notes of all admissions to a single hospital who had been given the diagnosis over a period of around 15 years. From these, the authors selected 43 (22 men and 21 women) who met both DSM-IV and ICD-10 criteria. Twenty-six had persecutory delusions, 12 had somatic delusions, 3 had delusional jealousy and 2 had erotomania. In line with other studies, the patients tended to be relatively old: the mean age at the time of the index admission was 51.8 ±12.6 years, and the mean age of onset was 46.9±13.2 years. Also in line with previous studies, 25 (58.1 per cent) were married or living with a partner.

It proved possible to reassess 33 of these patients on average 6.6±3.8 years later (3 had died and 7 refused to take part), corresponding to a period of 10.8± 4.7 years after the onset of the disorder. These patients were re-interviewed in person, where part of the examination included a structured psychiatric interview to verify the original diagnosis of delusional disorder and to document any new ones. Six of the 33 patients (18.2 per cent) were found to have developed schizophrenia, diagnosed according to DSM-IV criteria. One further patient had experienced a schizo-affective (manic) episode. Almost all the patients who had undergone diagnostic shift had delusions of the persecutory type, but one had erotomania. The change occurred on average 7.68±4.7 years after onset, with the standard deviation indicating that the range was wide.

Marneros et al.'s (2012) conclusion was that the diagnosis of delusional disorder showed a remarkable diagnostic stability. It should be noted, however, that, at 18.2 per cent, the rate of conversion to schizophrenia was actually at the higher end of the range of the studies reviewed by Kendler (1980), suggesting that the possibility that it is a form of low grade schizophrenia is no more ruled out than it was ever was.

If the relationship between delusional disorder and schizophrenia remains uncertain, its link with affective disorder seems if anything to have become stronger over time. The basis for the assertion that mood episodes up to and including major depression can occur in patients with the disorder, made from DSM-III-R onwards and also featuring in ICD-10, has never been very clear, although it may have reflected the influence of Munro. Nevertheless, all recent surveys of delusional disorder have found evidence for such an association. In the HADES study, for example, 9 of the 33 patients who were followed up had been hospitalized with an affective episode (not further specified). In another study (Maina et al., 2001), 23 of 64 patients who met both DSM-IV and ICD-10 criteria for delusional disorder were found to qualify for an additional lifetime diagnosis of major depression; the mood disorder preceded the onset of the delusional disorder in approximately one-third of cases. Grover et al. (2007) examined the case notes of 88 patients meeting ICD-10 criteria for delusional disorder and found that slightly over half had associated depression, and one had a previous history of mania. Similarly, de Portugal et al. (2011) found that 21 of 86 patients had experienced one or more episodes meeting criteria for major depression and two had a past history of hypomania.

Vicens et al. (2011) documented the association from another angle. In the course of recruiting patients for an imaging study of delusional disorder, they came across four patients in whom there was clear evidence of comorbidity with bipolar disorder; two of the cases are summarized in Box 3.3.

Box 3.3 Two Cases of Delusional Disorder Complicated by Bipolar Disorder (Vicens et al., 2011)

Case 1

A skilled worker in his twenties started to believe that his bosses and colleagues suspected he was involved in a theft at his workplace. He noticed his co-workers talking about him and giving him looks, and found that the settings of his machine were changed when he was not there. He eventually came to believe that his bosses were monitoring him with cameras and microphones. He moved to a different job and the symptoms stopped. Some months later, however, after a previous workmate appeared in the new workplace, they started again, and he became convinced that attempts were being made to poison him. The patient went on to change his job several times. When he did not work in his previous occupation he did not experience any symptoms. However, he was often attracted back by the high salary he could earn, and then the symptoms always returned.

Four years after his initial presentation the patient was admitted with a two-week history of expansive mood, irritability, decreased need for sleep, increased speech and disinhibition. He improved on treatment but did not persist with this and two years later had a further admission with similar symptoms.

Since then he has remained well on lithium and olanzapine. He works full time and has recently obtained higher qualifications. He has a long-term girlfriend who he lives with. The patient accepts that he has bipolar disorder but is convinced that this was caused by intentional poisoning.

Case 2

At the age of 33 a shorthand typist overheard a remark at work and realized that an event which took place six years previously, where she thought she was being suspected of cheating in an examination, had got back to her current place of work. From then on she started noticing her colleagues making comments about the matter. They would refer to her indirectly by using the name of a cheap brand of tampons or by repeating the slogan from a TV advert for a well-known Spanish department store. At one point someone at work commented 'Your husband wears glasses, doesn't he?', which she took to mean that the person was implying that her daughter was not her husband's. She was treated with olanzapine but remained symptomatic.

Ten years later she stopped all treatment. Her paranoid symptoms became worse, but then she became overtalkative and irritable. She started writing pages every day while listening to music and singing loudly. She was admitted and was noted to show pressure of speech and flight of ideas; she also described feeling that she was the best typist in the world and was unusually sexually attractive. She was treated with risperidone and slowly improved.

The final issue facing the modern concept of delusional disorder is one that has surfaced a number of times over the years, but has now reached crisis proportions. This is how to deal with the fact that most if not all of the subtypes of the disorder appear to have non-delusional counterparts. This led to DSM-IV taking a convoluted position where patients could be given a double coding. In DSM-5 this system has been replaced with one whereby patients are allowed to move in and out of the category of delusional disorder depending on the severity of the conviction of the belief. A war that is currently being fought out over this issue, and its battleground is body dysmorphic disorder.

On one side of the debate is Munro, who has continued to champion the view that delusional disorder with a dysmorphic delusion and body dysmorphic disorder are two completely separate entities. His argument, as set out in his 1999 book (Munro, 1999), hinges on the contrast between two patients he described in some detail. The first was a 26-year-old man who showed the features of delusional disorder, somatic type. He had a previous history of amphetamine and cannabis use, and more recently alcohol abuse. A knife fight had resulted in a facial disfigurement. He was referred for psychiatric assessment after an incident where he became angry after a surgeon had refused to operate and had attacked him and two clinic nurses:

> For about a year after the fight, he had led a relatively quiet life and did not appear to have any undue concerns. Then he started to feel that people were staring at him and mocking him, and he could not rid himself of this conviction. He was utterly preoccupied with this disfigurement and was convinced that people were laughing at him and talking about him because of it. He began to drink intermittently but heavily again, and his sense of tension only became worse. No one had suggested that surgery would be beneficial and his belief that an operation would magically cure him seemed to develop alongside his delusions of reference ... [A]fter two weeks of treatment [with antipsychotics] his mood began to improve rapidly, his preoccupation disappeared and he stopped hiding his face. He began to socialize again and reported that he had much less need for alcohol. At one-year follow-up his improvement was maintained, he did not worry about his appearance and he had no desire for surgery.

This was contrasted with a case of body dysmorphic disorder in a 35-year-old single mother of three children:

> The patient was extremely anxious and insisted she was physically disgusting because of abdominal striae related to her three pregnancies. She had made repeated demands for cosmetic surgery over the previous two years, was furious at being denied this, and was initially resistant to psychiatric assessment. Finally she agreed because it had been suggested that the psychiatrist might recommend surgery on 'mental health grounds'. At initial interview she was agitated, dejected, angry and demanding. She was not interested in any psychodynamic investigation of her symptoms. However, following a fairly lengthy session it seemed reasonably certain that she was not deluded, she could be engaged in debate about her symptoms and she could even agree that they might seem unreasonable to others. She did not claim that other people could see the stretch marks when she was clothed but claimed that the marks kept her from normal activities such as swimming, and ruined her chance of ever remarrying. She said she would kill herself if she could not have reparative surgery ... Despite grumbling about side effects [of antidepressants] (which were not severe) she began to improve. Distress and preoccupation were diminished, although they did not totally disappear. After two years the patient, although still chronically disgruntled, was involved in paid work, had some degree of social activity and said 'There's no point in trying to get plastic surgery because I'll never be able to afford it.'

Munro (1999) did not see a convincing link between the two presentations. In the first case the dysmorphic belief was held with full conviction and there were marked delusions of reference. In the second, the degree of conviction was not fixed and referential ideas were not present. Also important for Munro was the fact that the first patient responded promptly to antipsychotic treatment whereas antidepressants helped the second. Somewhat more tentatively, he also suggested that certain premorbid personality features were often seen in patients with body dysmorphic disorder – he specified obsessive-compulsive traits – but were not typical of patients with delusional disorder.

Munro's nemesis is Phillips, who has built her case on empirical data which point to the delusional and non-delusional variants of body dysmorphic disorder being on a continuum. In one such study (Phillips et al., 1994) 100 patients with body dysmorphic disorder were divided into 52 with the delusional and 48 with the non-delusional form, based on careful questioning about whether they were or had ever been completely convinced about their supposed defect. Demographics, illness characteristics, co-morbidity, family history, chronicity and most measures of functional impairment failed to distinguish the two groups. The only significant difference was that the delusional patients had significantly lower educational attainment. Results were similar in a later study (Phillips et al., 2006), where the patients were assigned to delusional and non-delusional categories based on cut-offs on a scale for delusionality.

Nor did presence or absence of referentiality seem to be a reliable distinguishing feature. Phillips (2004) found this to be present in two-thirds of a series of patients with body dysmorphic disorder, making it unlikely that it could be restricted just to patients with the delusional variant. The pervasive nature of the phenomenon is illustrated in Box 3.4, which also shows that the ideas can sometimes border on the ridiculous.

Box 3.4 Referentiality in Body Dysmorphic Disorder (Reproduced with Permission from Phillips 2005a)

One reason BDD is so painful and embarrassing to many BDD sufferers is they think other people take special notice of – and even mock – their defect. If someone glances in their direction, they think they're being looked at in horror or with disgust – that the glance reflects the fact that their defect is repulsive. One man concerned about a minimal scar on his neck said, 'I know people are smirking at me when they see me. When I cross at a crosswalk I think people in cars are thinking, "I wonder what happened to him. Look how ugly he is."' Another man worried about mild acne said, 'When I go out, I think everyone's noticing it. I think they're thinking "What's that ugly thing on his face?" It would be like if you painted big red marks all over your face and then walked down the street. Everywhere I go I feel like a neon sign is pointing at my face!'

People with BDD usually think that others can see the defect, but what I'm discussing here goes beyond this … Benign events in the environment unrelated to the person – or events that are related to them but have nothing to do with the supposed defect – are interpreted as referring to the flaw in a negative way. About 60 per cent of the people in my studies have had such experiences – for example, thinking that others are staring at, talking about, or making fun of how they look. About half of them think that other people *probably* are taking special notice of them, and about half are *completely convinced* of this. Some use the term 'paranoia' to describe their experience.

This was a serious problem for Jennifer, who left her car in the middle of a traffic jam because she thought other people were horrified by her skin. When she walked down the street, she believed that people stared at her skin and thought, 'That poor girl – look at her skin. It looks terrible!' When she entered a restaurant she believed the acne and marks distracted people from their meals, and she could eat out only if she hid in a booth in the restaurant's darkest corner. Even then, she had to look down at the menu while ordering her food so the waitress couldn't see her face. At work she thought co-workers were laughing at her behind her back. Because of this, she often left work in the middle of the day and eventually quit her job.

Conversations may be erroneously interpreted to refer to the person with BDD. 'Whenever people talk about shaving or beards, I think they might be referring to my beard,' Bart told me. 'They're really mean.' Some BDD sufferers think others can see the defect from impossibly long distances. One man thought that other people could see his minimal acne from 20 feet away, and Jennifer believed hers was visible from 50 feet. A man who sang in a choir thought the entire audience could see a small scar on his neck … Sometimes this referential thinking is more unusual. Jane thought that other people stared at her nose through binoculars. Another thought that as she walked by other people, they said 'She's ugly', or muttered 'Dog!' under their breath. When Alex was a child, he thought his mother left the table during meals because he was so ugly. 'This happened more often as I got older and uglier,' he said.

The final nail in the coffin for Munro's argument is that treatment trials have uniformly failed to support the view that delusional and non-delusional body dysmorphic disorder patients respond differently. Phillips et al. (2004) were able to find six trials of antidepressant drug treatment carried out by her and others, all of which found that the response was similar in both groups. In another study (Phillips, 2005b), she randomly assigned 28 patients to pimozide or placebo in addition to antidepressant treatment (fluoxetine). The strategy was not found to be effective and there were no hints of a better response in the delusional compared to the non-delusional patients.

Conclusion: Is Delusional Disorder Any More Likely to Survive than Paranoia?

Kraepelin's attempt to establish paranoia as a disease entity failed, undermined by an early attempt to discredit it and then a gradual descent into diagnostic chaos. But by then it had become a construct that refused to go away and, as delusional disorder, it now seems stronger than ever, supported by a substantial body of evidence indicating that patients showing the requisite clinical features exist and cannot be easily assigned to other diagnostic categories. But for all this, it remains a troubled category which may have a structural fault running through it.

Some of delusional disorder's troubles may be more apparent than real. The possibility that it is just a mild form of schizophrenia running a benign clinical course may not have been laid to rest, but seems unlikely to be the answer, if for no other reason than it shows what appears to be at least as strong an association with affective disorder. After all, if delusional disorder were simply a variant of schizophrenia, why would it be punctuated by episodes of major depression (and mania) in some patients? Of course, the same argument can also be levelled against delusional disorder being an unusual presentation of major affective disorder: if this were so, why do nearly a fifth of patients go on to develop schizophrenia?

In contrast, the question of how to reconcile the concept of delusional disorder with the undoubted existence of non-delusional forms of most or all of its subtypes remains seriously vexed. With Phillips having beaten Munro hands down, the currently favoured option is that the two presentations are on a continuum. Unfortunately, there is a problem with this proposal: if the arguments made in the last chapter are correct, then the abnormal belief in the non-delusional variant takes the form of an overvalued idea. This would then mean that overvalued ideas are on a continuum with delusions. Although such a view might be attractive to some, it should not be forgotten that accepting it also means accepting that some, perhaps the majority of patients with anorexia nervosa should be considered deluded. This is not a psychopathological position that seems likely to be adopted any time soon.

A radical solution might be to remove body dysmorphic disorder from the category of delusional disorder altogether; there would then be no delusional cases of this disorder, just as there are no delusional cases of anorexia nervosa. This is a position that has been argued for by de Leon et al. (1989) and it is something that the present author would have no difficulty accepting. The problem with taking such an approach is that it begs the question of what to do about the other two somatic subtypes of delusional disorder. The central belief in the olfactory reference syndrome has been argued to show the characteristics of an overvalued idea in some cases (Begum & McKenna, 2011; see Chapter 2), but it is not clear that this holds true in all patients, and there is the additional complication that some of them also experience the smell they believe they are giving off. When it comes to delusions of infestation the problem is even more acute: the fact is that many patients with this disorder have beliefs that are difficult to understand as anything other than delusions. An example is shown in Box 3.5.

Box 3.5 A Patient with Delusional Disorder, Somatic Subtype with an Infestation Delusion (Author's Own Case)

A woman in her thirties was admitted with a 4-month history of various physical symptoms that had been investigated with negative results. Her brother had a diagnosis of schizophrenia and her mother had been treated for depression.

On admission she was noted to have a complex system of hypochondriacal beliefs. She believed that the fibroids she had previously been diagnosed with had affected her intestines, making them rotten and causing hairs to grow in them. She saw what she variously described as hairs, specks and tiny balls coming out of her mouth; and similar things in other bodily fluids and faeces. She felt she was infecting other people she came into contact with, causing them to have gastritis, rhinitis and sore throats. She also worried that these people would then infect other people.

She stated she was completely convinced that all this was really happening. She would wash many times to try and get rid of the infection from her skin, although this kind of behaviour came and went. She would also step back from people she came into contact with to avoid infecting them and would try to avoid them having contact with her skin, e.g. by wearing long sleeves.

Structured psychiatric interview revealed no other abnormal beliefs, and there were no referential ideas or delusions. There were no auditory or visual hallucinations. However, she described a sensation in her stomach which rose to her throat and was bound up with the appearance of the hairs/specks. She also sometimes noticed a rotten or metallic taste in her mouth. There were also perceptual distortions: when her symptoms were very bad she would notice that smells in the street seemed more intense. Sometimes it also seemed as if the light suddenly became dimmer.

She stated that her symptoms had made her somewhat depressed when they first started and she lost several kilograms in weight. However, she denied being currently depressed and she had few biological or other associated symptoms of depression. Objectively, her speech was coherent and flattening of affect, if it was present at all, was no more than mild.

All investigations including MRI scan were normal. Treatment with antipsychotics resulted in some short-term improvement – she stopped seeing specks in her secretions and her bodily sensations become less intense.

At follow-up three years later she was in essentially the same condition and no new symptoms had emerged. She continued to believe she was ill and saw the same specks in her urine etc. She stated that she was not depressed and there was no evidence she had been depressed at any point in the preceding three years. She continued to work at her usual level.

Finally, running through the history of delusional disorder like a kind of subtext is the issue of the presence of referential delusions. It often seemed as if Kraepelin was trying to make these a cornerstone of the diagnosis, and Munro also deployed them to shore up his argument that there were distinct delusional and non-delusional forms of body dysmorphic disorder. However, the evidence is clearly in favour of these symptoms not necessarily being present, even in otherwise unequivocal cases of delusional disorder – with the patient in Box 3.5 providing a good example. At most, therefore, they can only act as a kind of diagnostic marker for delusional disorder in the same way as first rank symptoms are a diagnostic marker for schizophrenia – if they are present they support the diagnosis but their absence does not invalidate it.

The Pathology of Normal Belief

Up to now, this book has been solely concerned with beliefs that are abnormal. They occur in people who mostly show other evidence of mental illness, and even when the belief is completely isolated, it can still be considered pathological on the time-honoured grounds that the person concerned seeks help for it (or others seek help for it on his or her behalf). But strange ideas are by no means the exclusive preserve of psychiatry; there are many people who are not in any sense mentally ill who subscribe to all kinds of weird and wonderful, and at times flat-out wrong, beliefs.

The kind of irrational beliefs that immediately spring to mind in this context are those that from time to time grow up among groups of people, sometimes in small numbers, but occasionally coming to gain many adherents. The archetypal example here is cargo cults, the religious or quasi-religious movements which swept remote islands after they were visited for the first time by ships from the West (e.g. Lindstrom, 1993), or in more recent times, by planes (Raffaele, 2006). Something that seems on the face of it to be similar is the phenomenon of witch-hunts, both in their literal sense, as for example in the Salem and other witch trials of the seventeenth century, and in the figurative (and sometimes not so figurative) way the term continues to be used. Nor are science and medicine, whose practitioners pride themselves on their objectivity, immune to this kind of collective irrationality. It often seems as if psychiatry is especially susceptible – an easy target here is psychoanalysis, which dominated American psychiatric thinking for more than 30 years despite having absolutely no scientific basis and maintaining that anyone who did not accept its truths was exhibiting the unconscious defence mechanism of resistance. However, insulin coma therapy for schizophrenia and the indiscriminate use of frontal lobotomy provide grim examples from the other end of the therapeutic spectrum.

The problem with studying such group beliefs is deciding whether they are really false; this is ultimately a matter of opinion and history is littered with ideas that were initially ridiculed before going on to be universally accepted. In what follows, this difficulty is avoided by focusing on three examples where the beliefs concerned have been unequivocally proved to be wrong, or at any rate there are very good grounds for disbelieving them. An added bonus is that in each case attempts have been made to understand the psychological mechanisms that allowed the ideas to flourish, something that might provide some insights into the nature of more obviously pathological false beliefs.

The phenomenon of false or at least unusual beliefs in the non-mentally-ill population is not limited to those that are seen among groups of people. According to a long tradition in psychiatry, there are also people who are prone to more idiosyncratic irrational beliefs. Such beliefs were first noted in the relatives of patients with schizophrenia, who also showed peculiarities of speech and behaviour, leading to concepts like borderline schizophrenia, and more recently schizotypy and schizotypal personality disorder. Now, however, it is being argued that having minor or attenuated psychotic experiences is not just restricted to a small number of individuals who show definable psychiatric characteristics, but instead that they occur on a continuum of frequency and intensity across the population as a whole. Schizophrenia and psychosis then becomes a somewhat arbitrarily defined extreme end of this spectrum. This view also provides a potential window into the nature of delusions, one that is currently extremely influential.

Group False Beliefs

Millennial Cults

If evidence were needed that otherwise normal people can develop and hold on tenaciously to beliefs that are unquestionably wrong, one needs to look further than the movements which periodically arise over claims that the end of the world is coming. These are often referred to as millennial cults, since many of them revolve around the second coming of Christ, who it is believed will usher in the Millennium, a golden age of 1,000 years as prophesized in Revelations.

The social psychologist Festinger and two colleagues (Festinger et al., 1956) documented several examples of such movements. One early case concerned Sabbatei Zevi, an ascetic and student of the Cabala in what is now Turkey; in 1648 he announced to a small group of disciples that he was the Messiah, in accordance with a prophecy that such a figure would appear that year. He was banished by the religious establishment, but afterwards moved around the Near East attracting increasing numbers of followers from cities with Jewish communities, now proclaiming that the Millennium would arrive in 1666. The movement eventually became very large and many people sold their homes and possessions in anticipation of the return of the Jews to the Holy Land. At the beginning of the predicted year, he and some of his followers were in Constantinople hoping to depose the Sultan, something that was also supposed to occur in the days leading up to the Millennium. There he was arrested and imprisoned. This led to thousands of people gathering outside the place he was being held. Festinger et al. (1956) described what happened next:

> Finally, in an attempt to deal with the problem without making a martyr of Sabbatei, the Sultan attempted to convert him to Islam. Astonishingly enough, the plan succeeded and Sabbatei donned the turban. Many of the Jews in the Near East still kept faith in him. Explanations were invented for his conversion and many continued their proselyting, usually in places where the movement had not previously been strong. A considerable number of Jews even followed his lead and became Moslems. His conversion proved to be too much for most of his followers in Europe, however, and the movement there soon collapsed.

Festinger et al. (1956) also gave the more recent example of Miller, a farmer in New England who, based on an intensive study of dates in the Bible, came to the conclusion that the Second Coming would take place sometime between 1843 and 1844. He slowly built up a following, which ultimately became a mass movement. The most highly favoured date of 23 April 1843 came and went, leading to surprise and disappointment. However, the cult's followers were reassured by the fact that Miller's calculations allowed a date of up to 21 March 1844, and the fervour if anything increased. When this latter date also passed uneventfully, the discouragement was profound. Nevertheless, many followers were ready to attribute the failure to some minor error in the calculations, and they started to accept a new prediction of 22 October 1844. After no events materialized for the third time the movement disintegrated. Many of the believers were left financially ruined.

To explain this recurring pattern, Festinger et al. (1956) proposed that when an individual who holds a belief that is important to him or her is confronted with unmistakeable evidence to the contrary, an unpleasant state ensues, which they termed cognitive dissonance. One way to reduce the intensity of the state would simply be to give up the belief; however, if the commitment to it is strong, it is too painful to do this, and instead dissonance reduction is achieved by inventing ways of explaining away the inconsistency. Support for such a strategy is likely to be forthcoming from other individuals holding the belief, since they too are in the same state. However, even this might not be enough to remove the dissonance entirely, and so another approach is often employed, that of trying to convince other people that the belief is true. If a large number of people believe something, there will be fewer questions about whether it is actually true or not. In this way the individual emerges not only with his or her belief intact but also more convinced of the truth of it than ever. Of course, contradicted beliefs cannot be maintained indefinitely; sooner or later reality sets in and the belief is finally abandoned or at least stops influencing behaviour.

By chance, Festinger et al. (1956) had an opportunity to put their ideas to the test, thanks to an item they read in a newspaper about a small-scale movement that had sprung up prophesizing an imminent cataclysm (a flood). They decided to infiltrate the group and observe the unfolding events. As described in Box 4.1, the weekend immediately before the predicted date was marked by a series of disconfirmatory events. In line with the cognitive dissonance hypothesis, the first of these did not result in most of the group giving up their belief, but rather to them considering various possible explanations for the non-appearance of flying saucers to pick them up. The two leaders of the movement also became highly insistent that the flood was going to take place, preaching to anyone who would listen. Right up to the last moment, when the final predicted time for the aliens' arrival expired, the group remained fully convinced and ready to leave.

Box 4.1 A Field Study of an End-of-the-World Cult (Adapted from Festinger et al., 1956)

While working on their book about cognitive dissonance, Festinger and his co-workers by chance saw a press article about a suburban housewife, Mrs Keech (not her real name) who believed that a deluge would take place in the coming months and destroy a large part of the American continent. She had a long history of involvement in the occult and had begun receiving messages to this effect via automatic writing from beings from another planet (this was at a time when there was great interest in UFOs). The article indicated that she had attracted a small group of followers.

Festinger and some colleagues decided to start attending meetings of the group, posing as people who were interested in the occult and flying saucers and who had read the press report (they gave a detailed justification of why such a deceptive methodology was necessary, and were at pains to be as neutral as possible in the beliefs they expressed to the group). Mrs Keech herself made little active effort to convert the investigators, which may have been related to the fact that she had previously been visited by two mysterious people who told her not to further publicize the messages she was receiving. However, two of her main followers, a doctor and his wife, actively sought out followers, giving talks at church meetings and disseminating the text of her messages.

The messages had told the group that they would be picked up by flying saucers three or four days before the cataclysm and be taken to a place of safety, either on Earth or the aliens' home planet. They accordingly made active preparations for the event, and some gave up their jobs.

On the day when the group expected the flying saucers to arrive, a Friday, they removed all metal from their clothing. They also alerted the local press and television, which followed events over the weekend with bemused interest. When the predicted time for the arrival passed, the group was disappointed and considered various possible explanations for the non-appearance; they finally settled on it being a drill to test their preparedness. After this, the leaders engaged in strenuous teaching and explanation to anyone who was interested, including a variety of people who visited the house during this period. Several hoax calls purporting to be from representatives of the aliens were also taken literally by some of the members of the group. When the final allotted time came around, the group were again fully convinced and ready for the flying saucers to arrive. After a few more days and several more messages the group dispersed, although the main protagonists remained convinced that it had all been true.

The above case study, involving as it did individuals who could be considered self-selected for gullibility, might not represent a definitive test of the cognitive dissonance hypothesis. Nevertheless, a number of subsequent studies have tended to support the view that people who are placed in a situation of cognitive conflict tend to adjust their expressed views to reduce inconsistency (Draycott & Dabbs, 1998), although these studies are not without their critics (Chapanis & Chapanis, 1964). In any event, the term cognitive dissonance has gone on to enter the psychological lexicon (e.g. Harmon-Jones & Mills, 1999). Perhaps most importantly, it suggests that a formal cognitive mechanism may lie behind the way in which we often deceive ourselves when confronted with evidence that conflicts with our dearly held beliefs.

Witch-hunts

From the end of the fourteenth century, until the practice was progressively stamped out 400 years later, being denounced as a witch was a routine hazard to be faced in large parts of the Western world. According to Pavlac (2009), during this period millions of people suffered hate, guilt and fear, torture, arrest, and interrogation, and were sometimes executed, occasionally en masse. What social and psychological factors lay behind these witch-hunts cannot now be known with certainty. Some answers may, however, be found in a contemporary social phenomenon that seems similar in all respects, apart from the fact that the accused are not actually thought to have magical powers.

In the 1980s, allegations started to be made in America that organized sexual abuse of children was being perpetrated by adults who were devil-worshippers (Victor, 1993; Nathan, 2001). In many cases the precipitating event was a child who had started to show strange behaviour at school or in a kindergarten, or had symptoms such as painful bowel movements. On questioning, the child would describe horrific rituals, sexual abuse and even human sacrifices. Other children would be questioned and investigations would be mounted to find supporting evidence of a satanic cult. Adults involved in the care of the children, including parents, teachers and day care assistants, would be charged and not infrequently convicted and jailed. The first such case in 1983, involving a preschool in California, led to the longest and most expensive criminal trial in

American history. As in all other cases, none of the convictions were ultimately upheld (Eberle, 2003).

Satanic panic, as it came to be called, soon spread to other countries, with outbreaks taking place in Britain, Canada, Australia, New Zealand, the Netherlands and Scandinavia (La Fontaine, 1998). In two well-publicized cases in the UK (Jenkins, 1992), groups of children were forcibly removed from their homes in dawn raids by police and social workers, and alleged items of satanic paraphernalia were seized (example: a book with a goat on its cover). Both cases subsequently collapsed in court, with the judges deriding the lack of corroborative evidence, and making scathing comments about social workers being obsessed with satanism and subjecting children to repeated cross-examination, almost as if the aim was to force confessions out of them.

In the wake of this debacle, an anthropologist, La Fontaine (1998), was commissioned by the British government to investigate the two cases. She identified a number of reasons why 'concepts that seemed to be entirely mythical but which entailed the most fervent and unshakeable commitment' came to exert such a hold. These included the high levels of poverty, deprivation and abuse in the families concerned, but also the fact that many of the professionals involved had become convinced about the reality of satanic abuse from lectures they had attended and other sources. Another factor was the suppression of dissent in the relevant social services departments: 'In several cases, I heard an account of the extreme social pressure, up to and including complete ostracism, that had been exerted on those who doubted the diagnosis of satanic abuse in a case where their colleagues had accepted it.' Distrust between social service departments and police who were sceptical of the allegations was also considered to have played a part in strengthening the commitment of the former.

With these last two factors, La Fontaine (1998) was describing in all but name the phenomenon of groupthink. Janis (1983) used this term (whose Orwellian overtones were deliberate) to describe the 'shared illusions' that can arise when people with the same values work together in groups, particularly when they are under pressure or in a crisis situation. Groupthink is not simply a matter of powerful figures dominating and manipulating the other members of a group; instead, the leader is quite sincere in asking for honest opinions and the group members are not afraid to speak their minds. However, the presence of an atmosphere that values loyalty above everything else leads to the development of what Janis called a concurrence-seeking tendency, which prevents the individual members of the group from fully exercising their critical powers and openly expressing doubts. This causes all members of the group to stick with decisions even as it becomes clear that they are working out badly and may have morally disturbing consequences.

Janis (1983) identified various processes that contributed to groupthink, which fell into three broad groupings. *Over-estimation of power and morality* included the development of an illusion of invulnerability that was shared by most or all members of the group, which then led to excessive optimism and the taking of unacceptable risks. This was coupled with a belief in the group's inherent morality, which inclined members to ignore the ethical consequences of their decisions. *Closed-mindedness* showed itself in collective efforts to rationalize rather than reconsider assumptions, and in the adoption of stereotyped views towards the opposing group, such as their being too evil to negotiate with, or too stupid to counter risky attempts to defeat them. Finally, there were *pressures toward uniformity*: on the one hand, members of the group would start to 'self-censor' i.e. withhold their personal doubts from each other; on the other, if someone did openly dissent, explicit arguments, usually involving loyalty, would be brought to bear on him or her. Self-appointed 'mindguards' would emerge, who acted to protect the rest of the group from information that might adversely affect their shared views.

There have been few formal psychological studies of groupthink (for a review see Park, 1990). Instead the evidence in support of it rests mainly on Janis' (1983) analysis of a series of American policy failures that took place in different presidential administrations: the failure to anticipate the attack on Pearl Harbor (Roosevelt), the escalation of the Korean War (Truman), the Bay of Pigs Invasion (Kennedy) and the escalation of the Vietnam War (Johnson). In each case he was able to document a series of gross political miscalculations. That these examples reflected something more than just common or garden executive incompetence was further supported by two counter-examples where the group decision making functioned effectively: the Marshall Plan at the end of World War II and the Cuban missile crisis. These occurred in the same administrations as two of the aforesaid fiascos, and the latter involved almost the same group of officials as in the Bay of Pigs Invasion.

Was the great American foreign policy disaster of recent years, the Iraq War of 2003, a further example of groupthink? A surprisingly strong argument that it played a role has been made by Badie (2010). Among other things, she cited its explicit moral dimension, the Bush administration's overoptimism about the long-term consequences of regime change, and the famous 'stovepiping' of intelligence as an example of mindguarding.

Conspiracy Theories

Two years after the September 11 attacks on the World Trade Center, a senior British politician and ex-government minister wrote a comment piece in a national newspaper (see www.theguardian.com/politics/2003/sep/06/september11.iraq). In this, he noted that the scrambling of fighter planes in response to the hijacking of the four aircraft had been slow, and he wondered whether US air security operations had been deliberately stood down, perhaps as part of a neoconservative plan for the United States to seize control of the Arabian Peninsula. The US government angrily denied his allegations and it seems safe to assume that he did not endear himself to the leaders of his own party in Britain, which had been one of the few countries to support America in the invasion of Iraq.

Such is the power of conspiracy theories. Defined in a seminal essay by Hofstadter (1966) as belief in the existence of a 'vast, insidious, preternaturally effective international conspiratorial network designed to perpetrate acts of the most fiendish character', they vary considerably in their plausibility. The idea that John F. Kennedy was assassinated as part of a plot involving the CIA, Cuban counter-revolutionaries, the Mafia, the Russians or some combination of these, has been extremely tenacious over the years, and for a time was the official view following an acoustic analysis of the shots fired (the evidence was subsequently discredited). Rather more improbable are the beliefs that astronauts never landed on the moon; that Marilyn Monroe and Princess Diana (and sometimes also Princess Grace of Monaco) were murdered by various interested parties; that the US government was complicit not just in 9/11 but also in Pearl Harbor; that the existence of UFOs is known about and is being covered up; and that various secret societies from the Illuminati to the Bilderberg group control all the governments of the world. A conspiracy theory advocated by the British ex-sportscaster, David Icke, combines the last two themes, maintaining that the world has been secretly conquered by giant reptilian aliens.

Despite the fact that conspiracy theories require more than a little suspension of disbelief, the public appetite for them seems insatiable. The Kennedy assassination has spawned a never-ending series of books, as well as a successful Hollywood film. *Loose Change*, an internet documentary which argued that the 9/11 attacks were really carried out by the US government, has been watched by millions of people (Monbiot, 2007). Even David Icke's alien reptile theory does not lack for supporters (Barkun, 2013). Nor is it just the ill-informed or gullible who subscribe to them. In a book on the subject, Aaronovitch (2010) described how the writer and Washington insider Gore Vidal firmly believed that President Roosevelt had had advance knowledge of Pearl Harbor. He also quoted a fellow journalist as saying, 'I long ago accepted that in any gathering of five otherwise sensible people, there will probably be at least two who sincerely believe Diana was murdered.'

Knowledge of the psychological processes that lead people to believe in conspiracy theories is scanty. Most attention has been paid to personality factors, where studies suggest that there may be core of truth to the popular view of such individuals as being anti-establishment, easily influenced and with a deep interest in new-age cults and other minority beliefs. In support of this, a study by Goetzel (1994) found that people who thought that it was likely that President Kennedy had been killed by an organized conspiracy rather than by a lone gunman also showed a significant tendency to express agreement with nine other conspiracy theories. Other studies have found that belief in conspiracy theories is positively related to attitudes like openness to experience and political cynicism (see Swami & Coles, 2010).

Another psychological process that has been suggested invokes the role of so-called heuristics in thinking – a variety of mental shortcuts or rules of thumb that people tend to employ when they have to make decisions instead of properly weighing the evidence. The heuristic that has been considered to be most relevant to conspiracy theories is the proportionality bias, the tendency to consider that important events must have important causes. Brotherton (2015) vividly illustrated this principle in the following way. First he noted the mass of conspiracy theories that followed in the wake of the assassination of John F. Kennedy. He then turned to the assassination attempt on Ronald Reagan by John Hinckley, Jr, which had less public impact by virtue of being unsuccessful:

> The official story has it that Hinckley was mentally ill, and the shooting was a desperate attempt to impress the young actress Jodie Foster. He had pursued her for years, stalking her and sending her letters. Eventually, influenced by the film *Taxi Driver*, which starred Foster and featured the character Travis Bickle (played by Robert de Niro) planning to assassinate a U.S. senator, Hinckley decided the best way to impress Foster would be to kill the president ...
>
> Conspiracy theorists, on the other hand, would have us believe ... Well, actually there are hardly any conspiracy theories about Reagan's assassination.

The same author (Brotherton, 2013) reviewed four studies that examined the role of proportionality bias experimentally, using the example of a fictitious assassination attempt on a leader. Three found that subjects were more likely to attribute the event to a conspiracy if the president was killed or if the attempt led to a war, than if he survived or there were only minor consequences (McCauley & Jacques, 1979; Leman & Cinnirella, 2007; LeBoeuf & Norton, 2012). However, the fourth study, carried out by Brotherton himself, which used the scenario of a terrorist attack on an office building with small, medium or large numbers of casualties, failed to replicate the finding.

Neither of these approaches explains what is arguably the most important feature of conspiracy theories, the way in which their supporters blithely dismiss any arguments to the contrary, often citing them as further evidence of the establishment cover-up. But perhaps this feature of conspiracy theories does not need to be explained. In his book *Irrationality: The*

Enemy Within, the psychologist Sutherland (1992) systematically reviewed a large body of experimental findings which laid bare the way in which we all routinely distort evidence, draw the wrong inferences from data, are inconsistent in applying them and ignore anything that conflicts with our preconceived notions. Of the many studies he cited, one gives an idea of the scale of the problem. Lord et al. (1979) selected two groups of university students who were either proponents (N=24) or opponents (N=24) of capital punishment, based on their responses to an earlier questionnaire. The subjects saw, in random order, summaries of the results of four fictitious studies of murder rates, two of which provided evidence for the death penalty having a deterrent effect and two of which provided evidence against it. The subjects also saw critiques of the imaginary studies, which gave details of the research procedure, included tables and graphs of the findings, mentioned alleged criticisms that had been made by other researchers and even listed some of the fictitious authors' rebuttals of these. After reading all the material, the subjects were asked to rate the quality of the studies. Despite being exposed to identical evidence, they rated the studies that were in accordance with their existing views as being significantly more convincing and methodologically sound than the ones that contradicted them. Some of their comments are shown in Table 4.1. In a way reminiscent of cognitive dissonance, the subjects who were originally pro-capital punishment also reported that they were even more in favour of it at the end of the study, and those who were against it reported that they were more against it.

Idiosyncratic Abnormal Belief

Schizotypal Personality Disorder

The idea that some members of the normal population show characteristics that are reminiscent of schizophrenia is as old as the disorder itself. For Kraepelin (1913a), it was mostly a matter of personality traits; among the relatives of patients one saw 'striking personalities, criminals, queer individuals, prostitutes, vagrants, [and] wrecked and ruined human beings'. Bleuler's (1911) emphasis was initially also on character and personality ('irritable, odd, moody, withdrawn or exaggeratedly punctual people'), although later he (Bleuler, 1924) included people who tended to be suspicious or held unusual views ('pursuers of vague purposes, improvers of the universe, etc.').

Kendler (1985) has described how, in America, these views gradually morphed into the concepts of ambulatory schizophrenia (Zilboorg, 1941) and pseudoneurotic schizophrenia (Hoch & Polatin, 1949). These diagnoses referred to individuals who could appear superficially normal, but underneath showed a tendency to confuse the real world with fantasy, and harboured feelings of omnipotence and engaged in magical thinking. There was no requirement for such individuals to be relatives of patients with schizophrenia; in fact, the idea of the disorder being hereditary was anathema to psychoanalytic psychiatry, which dominated thinking at the time. Nevertheless, what Kendler (1985) called the genetic tradition never quite went away and ultimately reasserted itself as Meehl's (1962) concept of schizotypy. This was a hypothetical inheritable trait that was continuously distributed through the population, which manifested itself in an inability to experience pleasure, as well as in an aversion to social interaction and importantly in perceptual and thinking disturbances.

The two crisscrossing themes finally came together in the DSM-III category of schizotypal personality disorder, the criteria for which have remained essentially unchanged in DSM-IV and DSM-5. Such individuals show abnormal ideas that fall short of delusions,

Table 4.1 Examples of Comments Made by Subjects about Studies That Supported or Went against Their Pre-existing Beliefs on Capital Punishment

Attitude to Capital Punishment	Subject's Comments on Prodeterrance Study	Same Subject's Comments on Antideterrance study
In favour	'It does support capital punishment in that it presents facts showing that there is a deterrent effect and seems to have gathered data properly.'	'The evidence given is relatively meaningless without data about how the overall crime rate went up in those years.'
Against	'The study was taken only 1 year before and 1 year after capital punishment was reinstated. To be a more effective study they should have taken data from at least 10 years before and as many years as possible after.'	'The states were chosen at random, so the results show the average effect capital punishment has across the nation. The fact that 8 out of 10 states show a rise in murders stands as good evidence.'
In favour	'The experiment was well thought out, the data collected was valid, and they were able to come up with responses to all criticisms.'	'There were too many flaws in the picking of the states and too many variables involved in the experiment as a whole to change my opinion.'
Against	'There might be very different circumstances between the sets of two states, even though they were sharing a border.'	'These tests were comparing the same state to itself, so I feel it could be a fairly good measure.'
In favour	'It seems that the researchers studied a carefully selected group of states and that they were careful in interpreting their results.'	The research didn't cover a long enough period of time to prove that capital punishment is not a deterrent to murder.
Against	'It shows a good direct comparison between contrasting death penalty effectiveness. Using neighboring states helps to make the experiment more accurate by using similar locations.'	'I don't think they have complete enough collection of data. Also, as suggested, the murder rates should be expressed as percentages, not as straight figures.'

Source: Reproduced with permission from Lord, C. G., Ross, L., & Lepper, M. R. (1979). Biased assimilation and attitude polarization: the effects of prior theories on subsequently considered evidence. *Journal of Personality and Social Psychology*, 37, 2098–2109.

including ideas of reference, magical thinking, suspiciousness and paranoid ideation. They also have experiences that fall short of hallucinations, for example recurrent illusions or sensing the presence of a force or person not actually present. Other features include odd communication, inadequate rapport, inappropriate affect, social isolation, and eccentric or peculiar behaviour. Social anxiety is also present in many cases.

Individuals with schizotypal personality disorder, while showing unusual traits, are not mentally ill in the strict sense of the term, and so the fact that they have abnormal ideas is of some interest. But what ideas do they actually describe? Do they show attenuated forms of delusions, as the DSM definition suggests? Or are their ideas more like the minority beliefs described in the previous section? Or are they something else again? As it turns out, answers to these questions are not easy to come by, mainly because despite the reams that have been written about schizotypal personality disorder there very little actual clinical description. There is also the complicating factor that when cases are described, Asperger's syndrome often seems to be at least as appropriate a diagnosis as schizotypal personality disorder. A good example is 'Wash before wearing', included in both the DSM-III-R and DSM-IV Casebooks (Spitzer et al., 1989, 1994). This described a man with a lifelong pattern of social isolation who talked in often irrelevant detail about routine aspects of daily life. He could recite from memory his most recent monthly bank statement, including the amount of every cheque made and the balance on any particular day. His affect was considered to be distant and somewhat distrustful. He spent excessive periods of time thinking about minor matters, for example whether the washing instructions on a new pair of jeans meant that they should be washed before wearing the first time or that they needed to be washed after each time they were worn.

Accounts culled from the rest of the literature on schizotypal personality disorder are summarized in Table 4.2. While it has to be said that they do not give a very clear picture, some conclusions can be drawn. Sometimes the ideas described are not beliefs at all, but appear to take the form of fears and superstitions, although decidedly odd ones. Others clearly fall into the category of shared minority beliefs, for example ideas about clairvoyance and witchcraft. Some of the beliefs, however, do genuinely appear to be idiosyncratic; these mostly appear to have grandiose themes and there are suggestions that they are not held with full conviction. Referentiality is also apparent, but whether this amounts to anything more than simple, albeit unusual, ideas of reference is uncertain.

The Psychosis Continuum

Over the last 15 years or so the concepts of schizotypy and schizotypal personality disorder have found themselves taking a back seat to another, simpler formulation of the relationship between psychotic symptoms and their alleged less severe variants. This is that delusion-like and hallucination-like experiences are distributed throughout the population as a whole, including in many people who are otherwise healthy. The person who is almost single-handedly responsible for this reconceptualization is van Os (e.g. van Os et al., 2000, 2009; Johns & van Os, 2001). As he and a colleague (Delespaul & van Os, 2003) put it in a debate on the question of whether or not Jaspers was right and delusions are distinct from normal beliefs:

> The process of delusion formation is not irreducible but instead can be traced to a multifactorial aetiology involving an interaction, over the course of development, between a range of cognitive and emotional vulnerabilities, social circumstances and somatic factors, all of which are distributed in the general population and all of which may impact independently on one or more belief dimensions. The prediction of this model is that delusional beliefs of patients are continuous with the beliefs of non-patients, a notion that is increasingly supported by empirical evidence.

The study that launched this concept was the NEMESIS study, a cross-sectional survey of a large sample of the Dutch population (van Os et al., 2000). People aged 18–64 living in private households were interviewed using a computer-assisted psychiatric diagnostic interview designed to be administered by trained non-clinicians, the Composite International Diagnostic Interview (CIDI) (WHO, 1990). This has a psychosis section which covers persecutory and other delusions, thought interference, auditory hallucinations and passivity phenomena. Positive responses are explored and rated in one of four ways: as a 'true symptom'; as being 'not clinically relevant' (the individual is not bothered by it and is not seeking help for it); as 'secondary' (only experienced after taking drugs or in the context of physical illness); and finally as 'plausible', that is, not a true symptom because there appears to be some realistic explanation for it.

Out of the 7,075 individuals who took part, 4,165 were not given any psychiatric diagnosis. Of these, 42 (1 per cent) had true delusions as rated on the initial screening interview and

Table 4.2 Abnormal Ideas in Published Cases of Schizotypal Personality Disorder

Case	Abnormal Ideas	Comments
'Clairvoyant' (Spitzer et al., 1989)	Felt for many years that she was able to read peoples' minds by 'a kind of clairvoyance that I don't understand'. Preoccupied by the thought that she had some special mission in life, but was not sure what it was. Self-conscious in public, and often felt that people were paying special attention to her, or that strangers crossed the street to avoid her.	Included in the DSM-III-R Casebook but not in the DSM-IV Casebook.
'Weird and oddly preoccupied' (Cadenhead, 2014)	Suspicious that his classmates were undermining his abilities and telling his instructors that he was 'a weird guy'. Believed his thoughts often came true. Believed that coins could predict the future. He had once flipped a coin and had predicted his mother's illness. Had long thought that he could change the outcome of events like earthquakes by thinking about them. Fascinated by ghosts, telepathy and witchcraft.	-
Untitled (McKenna, 2007)	As a child felt figures that she cut out of cardboard boxes looked at her. As an adult believed that pictures she drew and her collection of records had magical powers.	-
'Dennis' (Lenzenweger, 2010)	Frequently thinks (but does not believe) that neutral events have special relevance for him, e.g. that shopkeepers set up their window displays with him in mind.	Alternative diagnosis of Asberger's syndrome seems possible.
'Stephen' (Lenzenweger, 2010)	Sees trails of yellow, red and blue light following behind stars and feels that these colours have special significance for him, suggesting that his inner nature is 'astral'. Reluctant to go into banks because he feels he may be observed and worries that bank tellers might try to cheat him.	-
'Alice' (Lenzenweger, 2010)	Often feels that numbers, symbols and certain images are imbued a magical power of sorts, and alters her behaviour depending on the numerals in the date. Pays close attention to the expressions of people who pass her by; a smile on the face of a stranger is often taken to mean that he or she knows something about her, usually something undesirable.	Alternative diagnosis of Asberger's syndrome seems possible.
'Claire' (Lenzenweger, 2010)	Has an unusual ability to sense what will happen in the world that goes beyond simple intuition, something akin to a sixth sense. Feels she can influence events with her mind, e.g. that she can make a red light turn green, although denies that she really believes that she can do so. Small figurines and amulets she collects help her find her way through the world.	-
'Neal' (Millon et al., 2004)	When briefly arrested, stated, 'I've thought for some time they wanted to set me up', 'They kept looking at me from outside the cell, although they tried to hide it, so I know they were talking about me.' Believes that he can occasionally see the future in a visual form. Claims that he can sometimes see what is going on in other places and what might happen if he were to go there.	-

(continued)

Table 4.2 (continued)

Case	Abnormal Ideas	Comments
'Matthew' (Millon et al., 2004)	Sometimes fears that he is dead or nonexistent, feels more like a thing than a person. He is helped by 'mind messages'. He calls out to protective spirits, who answer his call, reaffirming his existence.	-
Henry (Kwapil & Barrantes-Vidal, 2012)	Preoccupation with the spirit world (shared with associates). Feels the world is full of magical signs and signals that most people aren't aware of. For example a street number for a clinic appointment indicated that his spiritual essence would be endangered. Senses the presence of spirits and occasionally sees auras around people or animals.	-
Tamara (Kwapil & Barrantes-Vidal, 2012)	Felt that other students at art college criticized her, laughed at her and stole her supplies. Concerned that customers and employees in jobs talked about her. Would become focused on people eating in the restaurant where she worked and wondered if this was providing her with special messages about the world.	-

confirmed in a subsequent telephone interview with a clinician. A further 240 (5.8 per cent) had delusions that were classified as not clinically relevant. Sixty responses (1.4 per cent) turned out to have a plausible explanation. Only one participant had delusions that were rated as secondary. Findings were broadly similar for hallucinations, with 16 (0.4 per cent) having true, clinician-rated hallucinations and 137 (3.3 per cent) falling into the not clinically relevant category.

All types of delusion and hallucination rating were more common in the 2,910 individuals who were diagnosed with any form of mental illness. This was despite the fact that only 26 of these were given a diagnosis of schizophrenia or another form of non-affective psychosis. When the rates in these individuals were combined with those in the 4,165 individuals with no psychiatric diagnosis, 17.5 per cent reported at least one true or not clinically relevant delusion-like or hallucination-like experience. This was clearly a much higher prevalence than that of schizophrenia itself – 50 times greater according to van Os et al. (2000) – although this was based on a low estimate of the prevalence of the disorder of 0.4 per cent.

The NEMESIS study was by no means the first study to find evidence of psychotic-like experiences (PLEs) in healthy individuals. In fact, the earliest example seems to be a survey that was carried out by the British Parapsychological Society at the end of the nineteenth century (Sidgwick et al., 1894), and Linscott and van Os (2013) were able to find 61 more carried out between 1950 and 2010. One of these studies is of particular interest since it used an adaptation of the delusions section of the PSE. Verdoux et al. (1998) asked individuals visiting their general practitioners to fill in a self-report questionnaire, the Peters Delusions Inventory (PDI) (Peters et al., 1999). The PDI keeps closely to the original format of the PSE questions, although the questions are typically prefaced by the statement, 'Do you ever feel as if …'. Sixty-nine per cent of 462 subjects who did not have any known psychiatric history reported feeling that there were people around who were not who they seemed to be, and 42 per cent had noticed people dropping hints or saying things with double meanings. Rates were also substantial for experiencing telepathic communication (47 per cent), believing in the power of the occult (23 per cent), being persecuted in some way (25 per cent) and being especially close to God (21 per cent). Smaller numbers endorsed items about there being a conspiracy against them (10 per cent), being chosen by God (8 per cent), being like a robot or a zombie (9 per cent) or having an electrical device influencing their way of thinking (5 per cent).

Can it really be that up to two-thirds of the population at large experience something akin to delusions of reference and nearly half believe they are in telepathic communication with other people? Verdoux et al. (1998) were dismissive of the possibility that the participants in their study might simply have misunderstood the questions in the PDI, even though this is a well-recognized problem with self-report questionnaires (e.g. see David, 2010). It is true that more safeguards against this possibility were built into van Os et al.'s (2000) study – positive responses were classified as 'true', 'not clinically relevant', 'plausible', etc., and in some cases follow-up interviews were carried out – but even this may not have been enough to eliminate the possibility of misunderstandings altogether. This is because of a study carried out by Kendler et al. (1996) on a large community sample similar to that of the NEMESIS study. Individuals in this study who screened positive on the CIDI psychosis items were re-interviewed by a clinician. It was found that a substantial number of the responses that had been rated as 'possible, at least a suspicion of psychosis' or as 'probable or definite' psychotic symptoms were not actually psychotic-like in any meaningful way. Examples included culturally sanctioned beliefs such as in magic or witchcraft, what the author called isolated ideas of reference, and seeing a ghost or a recently deceased relative. CIDI items assessing common persecutory themes and thought transfer-like experiences were found to perform particularly poorly, being frequently misunderstood by the respondents and misinterpreted by the interviewers.

The issue of what might be termed the authenticity of PLEs was investigated further by Landin-Romero et al. (2016), in a study that also tested another prediction of the continuum proposal, that PLEs would be more frequent in individuals who were at increased genetic risk of schizophrenia. Forty-nine adult siblings of patients with schizophrenia and 59 matched individuals with no history of major mental illness in first-degree relatives were interviewed using the computerized version of the Diagnostic Interview for DSM-IV (C DIS-IV) (Robins et al., 2000), which like the CIDI is designed to be administered by trained non-clinicians (although in this case the interviewers were psychologists). Similarly to the CIDI, positive responses to psychosis items are explored and then rated as, 'plausible' (do not represent a psychiatric symptom because they have a real basis) or 'implausible' (represent a psychiatric symptom); in some cases whether the symptom occurred in relation to alcohol or drug use is also recorded.

Those who endorsed any of the C DIS-IV psychosis section questions, irrespective of whether their responses were considered rated as plausible, implausible or drug-related, were invited for a follow-up interview where the experiences were explored in depth using the PSE. These were then classified into one of five categories following a slightly modified version of the system used by Kendler et al. (1996): *misunderstood*, i.e. the individual was not describing anything that could be considered psychotic-like; *realistic*: for example, real persecution or harassment (also included here were the experience of hearing one's name being called in circumstances where it could actually happen such as crowded places, and non-pervasive simple ideas of reference such as transiently thinking people may have been talking about you when you enter a room); *light*: unusual experiences, usually occurring rarely, that raised no suspicion of psychosis; *drug related*; and finally *possible or probable psychotic symptom*. There was also an *unclear* category for experiences where there was insufficient information to form a judgement but the available information raised little question of psychosis being present.

Seventeen (34.7 per cent) of the non-relatives and 22 (37.3 per cent) of the relatives responded positively to one or more of the psychotic questions in the interview; this difference was non-significant. It proved possible to re-interview 30 of these participants (17 relatives and 13 non-relatives) with the PSE. Around two-thirds of the symptoms described in both groups fell into the realistic misunderstood or light categories. Under the heading of realistic were several examples of people who described noticing strangers looking at them because of the genuinely unusual appearance they had at the time (one was a DJ and an artist and liked to wear unusual clothes; another had long hair). Several gave credible accounts of people in their social group gossiping maliciously about them, or an ex-partner engaging in a hate campaign, or a colleague at work telling tales to their superiors, or a boss spying on them as part of a drive to identify which staff to fire. Some the more unusual examples in this category were the following:

> A woman had worked for a time in a totalitarian country. There was an official whose job was explicitly to check up on foreigners, and she used to see him following her to the supermarket. She wondered if he was also spying on her in other ways.
>
> A man who lived in a small town believed people thought he was gay, because he was unmarried and travelled a lot with another man (who was actually his brother). He knew people discussed this in the local bar, and they had openly said things to him about it.
>
> A man carried out some repairs for another person and they had a disagreement, during which the other person, who was a drug dealer, pulled a gun on him. Afterwards he noticed a certain car was often nearby when he was out and thought the person might be following him.

A frequent response for experiences classified as light was sensing the presence of relatives shortly after their death. This could take the form of a sensation of being touched by the person, or feeling a breeze, or in one case seeing a light crossing the room. For two years after the death of a relative, one participant also regularly smelt the bandages and medicines associated with his last days. Two subjects reported fleetingly smelling oranges or food cooking when there was no obvious cause for this. Also rated here were presumptively hypnagogic/hypnopompic experiences, such as a patient who occasionally felt paralysed for a few seconds when trying to relax, and another who felt a hand touching her on the shoulder when she was lying in bed and once had the impression that someone had got into bed next to her. One subject described the symptom of pareidolia: up to the age of 14 she used to see faces of animals and people in trees and buildings. Another had had the rare but entirely non-psychotic experience of seeing his life flash in front of his eyes when he was mountaineering and fell.

Misunderstood and drug-related categorizations were uncommon, and most of the remaining experiences fell into the possibly or probably psychotic category. Some examples of these are shown in Box 4.2; it can be seen that while a number were highly reminiscent of psychotic symptoms, others were less so, and instead resembled the kind of paranormal experiences that many people claim to have had. Once again, there was no obvious difference in the frequency of these experiences between the relatives and the non-relatives.

Box 4.2 Examples of Possible/Probable Psychotic-like Experiences in Individuals with and without a Family History of Schizophrenia (Landin-Romero et al., 2016)

a) Non-relatives

Around four years previously, he seemed to anticipate what people were thinking. When he asked the other person, he or she agreed. He knew things about them, e.g. that they had lost their job or had broken up with their girlfriend. Also 'clairvoyance' – he would suddenly understand something scientific, e.g. astronomy or engineering, without reading anything. When he checked in books it would be true.

He used to hear voices in the machine room superimposed on the noise. Two to three people, he couldn't make out the words. It happened early in the morning and late at night when there was no-one around. At first he thought it was a radio, but this wasn't the explanation. He and his co-workers used to discuss what was going on. Believes it was due to the fact that sound bounces off the walls to the extent that it can still be heard years later, even 30–50 years later. It's a natural phenomenon, not ghosts, etc.

She was not sleeping well because she was working nights. One evening while she was watching TV she suddenly she saw one of her workmates on the sofa next to her. It was a solid figure wearing a dressing gown. Without saying anything the person stood up and walked out of the room. The next day the friend confirmed that she was wearing the dressing gown concerned.

Two or three times a year she feels a strange sensation when she is about to touch something or someone, 'almost like a warning not to touch'. A physical sensation, lasts a second or two. She thinks that it is her grandmother who is guarding her.

Occasionally feels like his skin crawls and his hair stands on end and he shivers. It makes him wonder if the place he is in at the time is haunted, or someone died there. It could be something natural, but 'there's something there', i.e. something supernatural.

b) Relatives

After an acrimonious divorce 13 years ago, he became afraid of the possibility of his ex-wife getting her friends to beat him up. He took to walking down the middle of the road rather than on the pavement. From time to time he would see acquaintances on the street and knew they were talking about him. He felt criticized by everyone. He started confronting people about talking about him and then he would have to apologize when they denied it. Was convinced it was real at the time.

While he is out, on the street or in cars, or in social situations, he notices that girls look at him admiringly. As a result of this, men look at him enviously. The girls look at him and then they talk to each other about him. He has had arguments and fights with some of their boyfriends because of this.

Between the ages of 18 and 20, he felt that everyone was laughing at him because of his appearance (skinny and tall). In supermarkets he felt people looked at him and thought he was slow. He felt people sometimes followed him and felt frightened and in danger. At this time he was depressed and lacking confidence; he also lost weight, slept excessively and described loss of libido and irritability.

Once, as a child, she was looking at a photo of herself, and it looked like her lips were moving. It lasted more than half an hour. She talked to her mother about it who reassured her. It has never happened again.

> At the age of 6–7, she thought all her family was against her. She thought they were doing things on purpose, like not including her in a photo. She wondered if they were robots, if her real family had been replaced. It was a stressful period. Disappeared after some months.
>
> Once, as a child, he was watching TV there was a 'flash' in his head and he saw his father's car in an accident. It was very vivid. He had a similar experience as a teenager. Both times his father had in fact had an accident and the details in the 'flashes' were correct.

Conclusion: Does Normal Irrational Belief Help Us Understand Delusions?

Delusions, Jaspers (1959) argued, are qualitatively different from normal beliefs. He also implied that they are different from the kinds of irrational beliefs that people who are not mentally ill sometimes develop. An alternative narrative also exists, that Jaspers was wrong and delusions are simply one end of a spectrum of unusual beliefs seen in the population as a whole. The findings reviewed in this chapter have something to say about both these positions.

Psychology has done an admirable job in exposing how hopelessly irrational we all are almost all of the time, and it has also managed to make significant inroads into understanding why this is so. However, the hope that the false beliefs which lie at the heart of millennial cults, witch-hunts and conspiracy theories might have something to do with delusions is a mirage. This is because, unlike delusions, such beliefs are invariably (a) shared and (b) impersonal – they are held by groups of people and focus on events that concern all of them. Certainly, these beliefs are held with conviction, even fervour, and it is also true that they are characteristically immune to compelling counter-evidence. However, this is simply part of the human condition, something that was noted by Jaspers (1959), but actually goes back at least as far as to Francis Bacon writing in the seventeenth century, who was quoted approvingly by both Lord et al. (1979) and Sutherland (1992):

> The human understanding when it has once adopted an opinion draws all things else to support and agree with it. And though there be a greater number and weight of instances to be found on the other side, yet these it either neglects and despises, or else by some distinction sets aside and rejects, in order that by this great and pernicious predetermination the authority of its former conclusion may remain inviolate.

In Chapter 2, it was concluded that there are strong grounds for thinking that delusions in major affective disorder lie on a continuum with non-delusional but still pathological depressive cognitions or unfounded ideas. It seems only natural to suppose that corresponding lesser forms of non-affective delusions should also exist. The rise of this view over recent years has been spectacular, and it is now commonplace to see research articles reporting findings on the 'extended phenotype' of schizophrenia, i.e. not only those who meet diagnostic criteria for the disorder but also individuals who report having psychotic or psychotic-like experiences. However, the evidence in support of the continuum theory has an Achilles' heel: the nature of the PLEs that healthy subjects show has rarely been examined in detail. When attempts are made to do this, it turns out that quite a lot of what is being described is frivolous. No one would seriously argue that transiently feeling that people might have been talking about you when you walk into a room, or believing in the paranormal (which huge numbers of people do, to judge by the popularity of books and television programmes on the subject), or being prone to pareidolia or hypnagogic phenomena has anything to do with psychosis.

But at the same time, this is not the whole story. Some otherwise healthy people – it is impossible to say how many, but probably at least a third less than the 6.8 per cent found by van Os et al. (2000) – do have ideas that genuinely look like attenuated forms of referential and propositional delusions. Some of these individuals may have schizotypal personality disorder and some of them may have had major depression at the time they were having the experiences (there was evidence for both of these in the study of Landin-Romero et al., 2016), but almost certainly not all of them. Whether these symptoms occur with enough frequency for the continuum view to remain tenable is a question that only time, and studies that are an order of magnitude more critical than most of those that have so far been carried out, will tell.

Chapter

The Psychology of Delusions

5

Clinical approaches, from Jasperian phenomenology to van Os's continuum theory, can only go so far. There comes a point where they have to give way to attempts to identify the psychological abnormality or abnormalities that cause patients to experience delusions. The literature in this field is relatively rich, in the sense that several different lines of investigation have been pursued and methodological standards have generally been high. But it is also fair to say that it is very much a hotchpotch, with some more or less fortuitous empirical findings on the one hand, and on the other a clutch of theories that have been subjected to widely different amounts of testing.

The more or less fortuitous empirical findings grew out of a slowly dawning realization that schizophrenia is associated with cognitive impairment. Although it had been known since the 1930s that, as a group, patients with the disorder performed poorly on virtually any cognitive test they were given, it was only from the late 1970s onwards – coinciding with psychoanalytical psychiatry's fall from grace in America – that it became acceptable to view this as being due what it obviously was due to, the presence of varying degrees of general intellectual impairment. As further investigations were undertaken, it became clear that impairment was particularly marked in certain areas of cognition, including executive or frontal lobe function, long-term memory and sustained attention. If the disease process of schizophrenia could cause specific cognitive deficits, some of which are associated with damage to particular parts of the brain, might it be, it was wondered, that these deficits could also give rise to the symptoms of the disorder? The focus of attention quickly became executive impairment, and a whole industry sprang up devoted to drawing parallels between different clinical features of schizophrenia and the symptoms and signs of the frontal lobe syndrome (e.g. Seidman, 1983; Weinberger, 1988; Robbins, 1990; McGrath, 1991; Frith, 1992). As will be seen, however, delusions were not destined to yield to an analysis.

Even when it was at the height of its influence, the stranglehold of psychoanalysis over thinking about schizophrenia was not total and a few scientific approaches to delusions managed to eke out an existence. Since its fall many more have been proposed. Some of these continue to be rooted in the concept of a brain-based psychological dysfunction, but do not assume a simple one-to-one mapping between particular regions and symptoms; these are the so-called cognitive neuropsychological or cognitive psychiatric approaches. Others ignore brain localization altogether, and simply aim to discover a cognitive abnormality that is present in patients who are deluded. An important by-product of both these latter approaches is that the abnormal function is no longer constrained to being a deficit, as it is in neuropsychological theories, but is now free to take the form of hyperactivity, or altered processing of information in a system, or any of the various other ways in which cognitive psychologists are accustomed to thinking.

A convenient place to start a discussion of the psychology of delusions is with the neuropsychological approach, where the concepts are simple and straightforward. This then lays the groundwork for the somewhat more complicated cognitive neuropsychological approach. Only two proposals of this type are considered here; discussion of a third important approach is postponed to Chapter 7, partly because it is mainly devoted to delusions and delusion-like symptoms in neurological patients rather than those with psychiatric disorders, and partly because it needs a whole chapter to itself. Finally, the success or otherwise of some of the more important purely cognitive approaches is examined.

The Neuropsychology of Delusions

In 1980, Crow galvanized the world of schizophrenia research by arguing that the many and varied symptoms of the disorder showed a previously unsuspected underlying order. Specifically, he drew a conceptual distinction between positive symptoms, i.e. those that were characterized by the presence of an abnormality – such as delusions, hallucinations and formal thought disorder – and negative symptoms, where there was an absence or diminution of a normal function, such as lack of volition, poverty of speech and flattening of affect. Making such a distinction seemed to have deeper implications: for example, positive symptoms were characteristic of acute schizophrenia, which tended to be episodic and responded to treatment with antipsychotics, whereas negative symptoms were typically seen in chronic schizophrenia, where they were enduring and drug treatment was at best only marginally effective. This in turn suggested that there were two different pathological processes in schizophrenia, one reversible and perhaps neurochemical in nature and the other, which Crow (1980) speculated (wrongly as it turned out) might be related to the lateral ventricular enlargement seen in the disorder, which he and his colleagues (Johnstone et al., 1976) had recently discovered.

Two years later Andreasen and co-workers (Andreasen, 1982; Andreasen & Olsen, 1982) were able to show that, whatever the distinction between positive and negative symptoms meant aetiologically, it was valid at the clinical level – positive symptoms tended to correlate significantly with other positive symptoms but not with negative symptoms, and vice versa. True, there were some minor anomalies. One of these was that delusions and hallucinations appeared to be considerably more strongly associated with each another than with formal thought disorder. Another was that an uncommon symptom, inappropriate affect, did not correlate with symptoms in either category.

The true significance of these irregularities became apparent when Liddle (1987a) used a more sophisticated method for examining associations among multiple variables, factor analysis. He applied this to detailed ratings of the symptoms of 40 chronic schizophrenic patients with stable clinical pictures, and found that three factors emerged. Two of these were immediately recognizable as positive and negative symptoms: one had high loadings on auditory hallucinations, delusions of persecution and delusions of reference; Liddle termed this factor reality distortion. The other, which he called psychomotor poverty, loaded heavily on poverty of speech, decreased spontaneous movement, unchanging facial expression, paucity of expressive gestures, affective non-responsivity and lack of vocal inflection. The third factor was composed of various elements of formal thought disorder, plus inappropriate affect. Liddle termed this the disorganization syndrome.

The validity of Liddle's three syndromes is now widely accepted. Most subsequent factor analytic studies (see Andreasen et al., 1995; Thompson & Meltzer, 1993) have continued to isolate three factors; the small minority that have not have either tended to split the positive or negative factor in some not very intuitive way, or merely found additional factors corresponding to depressed or elated mood. Three studies using confirmatory factor analysis, which tests the goodness-of-fit of different models, all found that more than two factors were needed to satisfactorily account for the pattern of correlations among schizophrenic symptoms and that there was little to choose mathematically between three- and four-factor models (Brekke et al., 1994; Dollfus & Everitt, 1998; Peralta & Cuesta, 1994).

Just as Crow (1980) argued with positive and negative symptoms, the existence of three distinct constellations of symptoms in schizophrenia implies the presence of three different underlying pathological processes. Liddle (1987b) tested this prediction neuropsychologically. In 47 chronic schizophrenic patients, negative symptom and disorganization scores were found to be associated with poor performance on a number of different cognitive tests, with the pattern of correlations being somewhat different for the two syndromes. In contrast, reality distortion correlated with impairment on only one test (which measured figure – ground perception). For some reason, Liddle (1987b) did not actually include any tests of executive function in his battery, even though by then this had become the main focus of interest in neuropsychological schizophrenia research. However, this omission was put right in a subsequent study (Liddle & Morris, 1991), which used four executive tests. Once again significant correlations were found with negative symptoms and disorganization, but not with reality distortion.

The present author and a colleague (McKenna & Oh, 2005) reviewed the many further studies that have examined the associations among the positive, negative and disorganization syndromes and a wide range of cognitive test measures. The results are shown in Table 5.1. Both negative symptoms and disorganization were often, though by no means always, found to show significant correlations with impairment on tests of executive function, and also with tests of memory, language, visual and visuospatial function and even general measures such as IQ. However, only three studies found evidence for an association with reality distortion.

Even this minimal support for an association between reality distortion and cognitive impairment vanished in a meta-analysis examining the relationship between Liddle's three syndromes and executive function. Dibben et al. (2009) found that the pooled correlation between tests of executive function and reality distortion scores was +0.01 in 34 studies. In contrast there were small but significant pooled correlations with negative symptoms (-0.21 in 83 studies) and disorganization (-0.17 in 40 studies).

The conclusion is stark: while neuropsychological theories of negative symptoms and disorganization are possible, reality distortion, and so by extension delusions, cannot be explained in such a way. The lack of correlation between reality distortion and measures of general intellectual function like IQ also makes it unlikely that delusions could be associated with some as yet undiscovered aspect of neuropsychological function; general intellectual impairment would by definition also affect this unknown cognitive system. The only way that a neuropsychological deficit might be able to play a role in the development of delusions appears to be in the special case that it is merely one step in a more complicated chain of

Table 5.1 Neuropsychological Correlations with Positive, Negative and Disorganization Syndromes in Different Studies

	Reality Distortion	Disorganization	Negative Symptoms
Executive function			
Wisconsin Card Sorting Test		✓3✓19✓5✓22✓23✓6✓21✓18✓24✓9	✓12✓13✓4✓17✓24✓9
Verbal fluency	✓9	✓3✓9✓2✓16	✓3✓12✓13✓19✓4✓23✓16✓17✓9
Stroop test	✓10	✓3✓14✓22✓10✓26	✓3✓7
Trailmaking test (B)		✓3✓18✓22✓23✓9	✓13✓19✓4✓23✓9
Short-term and working memory			
Verbal (digit span)		✓18✓22✓4✓20	✓8✓21
Non-verbal (Corsi blocks)	✓1		
Working memory		✓23✓24	✓23
Long-term memory			
General memory		✓15	✓13
Verbal memory	✓12	✓1✓8✓18✓25	✓12✓13✓19✓17
Visual memory		✓12✓13	✓8✓13✓19✓17
Other		✓2	✓1
General intellectual function			
Full scale IQ		✓13✓19	✓13
Verbal IQ		✓8	✓8
Performance IQ			✓17
Other IQ		✓7✓8✓2	✓1✓2✓7
Miscellaneous			
Language		✓8	✓1
Visual/visuospatial function			✓11
Sustained attention		✓1✓18✓2✓21	✓19✓18✓2✓21

[1]Liddle (1987b); [2]Frith et al. (1991); [3]Liddle and Morris (1991); [4]Brown and White (1992); [5]Van der Does et al. (1993); [6]Bell et al. (1994); [7]Brekke et al. (1995); [8]Cuesta and Peralta (1995); [9]Himelhoch et al. (1996); [10]Joyce et al. (1996); [11]Cadenhead et al. (1997); [12]Norman et al. (1997); [13]Basso et al. (1998); [14]Baxter and Liddle (1998); [15]Clark and O'Carroll (1998); [16]Robert et al. (1998); [17]Mohamed et al. (1999); [18]Eckman and Shean (2000)Rowe and Shean (1997); [19]O'Leary et al. (2000); [20]Tabares et al. (2000); [21]Guillem et al. (2001); [22]Moritz et al. (2001); [23]Cameron et al. (2002); [24]Daban et al. (2002); [25]Pollice et al. (2002); [26]Woodward et al. (2003).
Source: McKenna, P. J. & Oh, T. (2005). *Schizophrenic Speech: Making Sense of Bathroots and Ponds that Fall in Doorways*. Cambridge: Cambridge University Press.

cognitive events. This idea forms the basis of the class of cognitive neuropsychological theories discussed in Chapter 7, but for the time being something beyond a simple deficit account of delusions seems to be required.

Beyond Neuropsychology: The Cognitive Neuropsychology of Delusions

Any theory that tries to explain delusions in terms of impaired neuropsychological function is, it seems, doomed to failure. But perhaps this is just a reflection of the rather simplistic approach to neuropsychology that has so far been taken. After all, not all of the symptoms of localized brain damage take the form of loss of function. One obvious example is fluent dysphasia; another is confabulation in patients with amnesia (a topic which is revisited in Chapter 7). The idea of mapping cognitive functions to discrete areas of the brain may also be too simple in another way – many specific neuropsychological functions are likely to depend on the joint operation of widely dispersed brain areas. As the network of regions involved becomes more complicated, the potential ways in which dysfunction might manifest itself might also become more varied, and it becomes possible to think about release from inhibition or lack of monitoring or some other consequence of failure of the normal interaction between modules making up a cognitive system.

This, at any rate, is the hope of cognitive neuropsychiatry. As described by two of its founders, Halligan and David (2001), this discipline aims to explain psychopathology in terms of altered function of normal cognitive mechanisms, based on the assumption that 'complex interactions between neural systems presumably underlie most psychological processes [and] no neuropsychological account of how the brain "works" would ever be complete without this cognitive level of analysis'. They also make it clear that alterations in the interactions between neural systems will result in something more than just impaired function: 'Psychological disturbances experienced by psychiatric patients are slowly coming to be understood in terms of disturbances – excesses as well as deficits – to recognized information-processing systems.'

For Halligan and David (2001) the paradigmatic example of how the cognitive neuropsychiatric approach can be applied to delusions was the Capgras syndrome, the belief that one's wife, husband or other family member has been replaced by an almost identical double, which occurs in patients with a range of neurological diseases as well as in psychiatric disorders like schizophrenia, and is discussed in detail in Chapter 7. Leaving this aside, they identified semantic memory as a promising area for a cognitive neuropsychology of delusions. They also felt that the concept of theory of mind might also be a good place to look, although not specifically in relation to this symptom.

Semantic Memory

Semantic memory is the store for all knowledge about the world. The concept dates back to a famous observation by Tulving (1972) concerning the two different ways in which the term memory can be used. On the one hand there is episodic memory or memory for events, i.e. memory for one's own individual happenings and doings, such as what one had for breakfast and who one met on holiday last year. On the other hand, everyone has a vast store of impersonal knowledge which, like episodic memory, is held outside consciousness but can be accessed into it when required. For Tulving, this impersonal knowledge was originally knowledge of the meaning of words, but he and others (Kintsch, 1980; Tulving, 1983) soon realized that the concept also applied to all other knowledge, from simple factual information such as knowing the capital of France or the chemical formula for salt, to abstract concepts such as truth and justice.

A cognitive system concerned with what we know to be factually true clearly has potential as a theory of delusions, specifically propositional delusions. This is particularly so when it when it is realized that a there is a recognized subdivision of semantic memory which holds one's knowledge about oneself. The most basic item held in personal semantic memory is one's name, but this type of knowledge extends to all kinds of personal data ranging from what one does for a living and where one lived at different times of one's life, to what kind of restaurants one likes to go to and which political party and football team one supports.

As befits a candidate for a cognitive neuropsychiatric theory, semantic memory is firmly anchored in regional brain function. This became clear only relatively recently, however, when Warrington (1975) described three patients whose unusual pattern of perceptual, language and memory deficits could be understood as a progressive breakdown of semantic knowledge. Subsequently semantic dementia, or the temporal lobe variant of fronto-temporal dementia, has become a well-established clinical and pathological entity (e.g. Hodges, 2007; Snowden et al., 1989). As described by Hodges et al. (1992) and Snowden et al. (1996), it typically starts with an inability to remember the names of people, places and things. The deficit is not restricted to naming, however, and patients also perform poorly when asked to give definitions of words, with their responses being grossly impoverished and often containing elementary factual errors. Although the patients complain that they 'can't remember anything', episodic memory remains intact until late in the course of the illness, and they are able to find their way around, keep appointments, and have no difficulty remembering day-to-day events.

Many studies (reviewed and meta-analysed by Doughty and Done, 2009) have documented that semantic memory is an area of impairment in schizophrenia. Of course, the fact that reality distortion is not associated with neuropsychological deficits in general makes it unlikely that there would an association between delusions and semantic memory impairment in particular, and this is exactly what was found by Mortimer et al. (1996) in a study using the Sentence Verification or 'Silly Sentences' Test (Collins & Quillian, 1969), where subjects have to indicate whether statements such as *Rats have teeth* and *Onions crush their prey* are true or false. The task is very easy and performance is measured in terms of speed of verification of the sentences. Fifty-three chronic schizophrenic patients showed no significant correlation between speed of verification and scores on a delusions scale.

On the other hand, a hint that semantic memory dysfunction in schizophrenia might involve more than just impairment came from a further examination of the findings from the same group of 53 schizophrenic patients by Tamlyn et al. (1992). As expected, the patients were found to be significantly slower at verifying the sentences than a group of 38 age-matched healthy controls. More interestingly, whereas none of the controls made more than two verification errors, 14 (26 per cent) of the patients made three or more errors, with 5 making them in large numbers (>10); these were often but not always in the direction of verifying false statements as true. Errors were seen particularly in patients with formal thought disorder, but also in a small number of patients who had clinical pictures dominated by florid delusions.

There were further hints in a study by Chen et al. (1994) with the title 'Semantic memory is both impaired and anomalous in schizophrenia'. They used a task in which the subjects had to decide, by pressing a button, whether or not a word displayed on a screen belonged in a particular semantic category. For example, the subjects would see the category *bird*, which on different trials would be coupled with exemplars such as *robin* (typical of the semantic category), *turkey* (atypical but still within the category), *penguin* (borderline), *aeroplane* (related but outside the category) and *bell* (unrelated). Twenty-eight healthy controls showed increasing response times as they moved from the typical to the atypical and the borderline exemplars, with response times then decreasing again progressively in the related and unrelated categories. Thirty-nine schizophrenic patients were found to be overall slower than the controls, but additionally their response times increased progressively up to the related but outside category, and only decreased again in the unrelated category. The same pattern was found when errors rather than reaction time were analysed. In this study, however, in contrast to that of Tamlyn et al. (1992), the apparent outward shift of semantic category boundaries in schizophrenia was not associated with any symptom.

The definitive study examining semantic memory in relation to delusions was carried out by Rossell et al. (1998). They used the Silly Sentences task but modified it in two ways. First, they made it harder, so that not only patients but also controls would make significant numbers of errors. This was achieved by including not only obviously true and obviously false sentences but also a third category of statements that could be true in some situations, for example *Leaves are red*. Secondly, they manipulated the emotional content of all three types of sentences so that some of them touched on common delusional topics. Accordingly, there were sentences with a violent or dangerous themes such as *Knives are dangerous* (true); *A cactus can bite* (false); and *Joy riders can return the cars they steal* (unlikely); those with themes associated with superiority, such as *Inventors are talented and clever* (true), *Scientists can turn grass blue* (false) and *Dentists can be talented artists* (unlikely); and those with a religious dimension, such as *Vicars work on Sundays* (true); *The bible is a car catalogue* (false); and *Monks are alcoholics* (unlikely). Other sentences had a political, sexual or health content. The predictions were that deluded schizophrenic patients would show more errors than controls, particularly when the sentences had an emotional content, and that they would tend to accept ambiguous sentences as true if they were congruent with their delusional ideas.

Sixty-three patients meeting DSM-IV criteria for schizophrenia or schizo-affective disorder were compared to 66 well-matched healthy controls. Both groups made small numbers of errors (<10 per cent) on the true and false sentences, but many more (>50 per cent) on the unlikely ones. The schizophrenic patients did not make more errors overall, and there were no marked differences between the groups with respect to emotional type. The crucial comparison concerned the relationship with the schizophrenic patients' delusions. To examine this, the patients' two to three most common past or present delusions were classified as persecutory, grandiose, political, religious, or involving relationships or bodily function, and any errors they made on the emotional sentences were rated as 'delusion congruent' or 'delusion incongruent'. An initial analysis showed that the patients made similar numbers of errors on emotional sentences that were congruent with and not congruent with their delusions. However, they also showed a small but significant tendency to incorrectly accept false statements (i.e. answering true to nonsense sentences) and incorrectly reject true statements (i.e. answering false to true and unlikely sentences). The findings are shown in Figure 5.1.

A reasonable interpretation of Rossell et al.'s (1998) findings might be that while deluded patients may show erroneous knowledge about the world in areas of semantic memory related to their delusions, this is subtle to the point of testing the limits of the technique used. However, it might be wrong to dismiss the possibility altogether. This is because another study has had quite similar findings. Laws et al. (1995) carried out a single case study (a respectable research strategy in neuropsychology) on a schizophrenic patient with a clinical picture consisting almost entirely of grandiose delusions. The patient was a 39-year-old man who believed he was a Baron, and that he was, or was about to become, a Conservative MP (and also manager of a football club). His general intellectual function was relatively

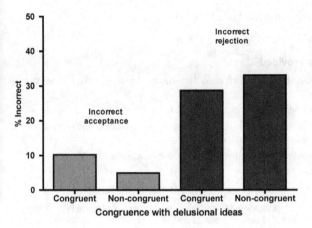

Figure 5.1 Schizophrenic patients' errors in sentence verification as a function of whether they were congruent with their delusions. The interaction term in the ANOVA was significant.
Source: Rossell, S. L., Shapleske, J. & David, A. S. (1998). Sentence verification and delusions: a content-specific deficit. Psychological Medicine, 28, 1189–1198.

well preserved (estimated premorbid IQ 107, current IQ 99), but, like many patients with schizophrenia, he showed mild to moderate impairment in executive function and long-term memory. More unusually, he also showed a moderately severe deficit in recognition of faces. For example, when presented with a series of 53 photographs of famous people (e.g. Marilyn Monroe, Nelson Mandela, Mother Theresa, James Dean), he named only 18, in comparison to mean of 39.6 in 20 age and premorbid IQ matched healthy subjects. Even when he recognized the faces as familiar without being able to name them, his knowledge about the people concerned was obviously impaired: he was able to give their occupation in 39 cases, but produced specific identifying information in only 19, and what he said sometimes contained gross errors, as shown in Table 5.2. The normal controls were at ceiling on these two aspects of the task.

Laws et al. (1995) noticed that many of the faces the patient named correctly were of politicians. When subsequently shown a new set of photographs of 34 domestic and international politicians (e.g. Anthony Eden, Dwight Eisenhower, Harold Wilson, Indira Gandhi, Ayatollah Khomeini), he correctly named 19/34 (55.9 per cent) of them, in contrast to 15/76 (19.7 per cent) of a set of famous people from other walks of life. As also shown in Table 5.2, the responses he gave in response to the names of the politicians (at least the British ones) were much richer in detail than for the non-politicians. At the same time, however, his descriptions showed a tendency to include fabricated material that was often highly unlikely, e.g. that David Owen, a prominent member of the Social Democratic Party, was also leader of the Scientologists and that the leader of the Liberal Party, David Steel, had stood in the Italian elections. The presence of such material was more frequent for the politicians than for the non-politicians (57 per cent vs 17 per cent).

This case could be considered nothing more than a curiosity – most patients with schizophrenia do not show marked impairments in familiar face processing, although another such patient has been reported (Shallice et al., 1991) – but it is intriguing that, in the midst of a marked deficit in semantic memory for people, the patient showed an island of preserved knowledge for British politicians, which also happened to be one of the themes of his delusions. Here, in line with what might be expected from a cognitive neuropsychiatric theory of delusions, some of the stored information also appeared to be corrupted.

Table 5.2 Laws et al.'s (1995) Patient's Knowledge about Famous People

A. General

Name	Information Provided
Marilyn Monroe	American actress I think. I wouldn't know if she was dead or alive, but I think she's still alive.
Elvis Presley	I think he's an American singer and musician, still alive.
John F. Kennedy	Former president who was killed in Dallas in 1963, killed by Oswald Mosley, it was tragic. I'm not sure if Mosley was found guilty or not.
Telly Savalas	'Ironside', he was bald, he played 'Ironside', detective, he was in a wheelchair.
Luciano Pavarotti	A ballet dancer I think.
Yasser Arafat	Don't know much about him, except that he's the Israeli Prime Minister.
Nelson Mandela	He's made a comeback recently, Kenyan leader, he won the Nobel Peace Prize, sharing it with someone else, he's been in prison as well.

B. Domestic politicians

Name	Information Provided
Margaret Thatcher	Ah, Mrs T, best Prime Minister in my lifetime, leader of the Conservative Party since 1979. Former MP for Finchley, she came from Grantham, you know. Married to a Dennis, a millionaire. She wrote to me, asking me to take the Plaid Cymru seat. We should not have got rid of her. I feel personally responsible for the demise of Mrs Thatcher because I voted against her in the second ballot. Now known as Baroness Thatcher, a member of the House of Lords.
John Major	I've met him in Huntington, he smiled at me, but his wife ignored me. Wrong choice as Prime Minister. Dubious whether he's suited to being an MP, never mind Prime Minister. He was chief secretary to the treasury before. Also foreign secretary for six months. Never even went to University.
David Steel	He was a famous leader of the Liberal party. Went on with David Owen to form the Alliance – SDP – Social Democrat Alliance. David Owen is now in Bosnia, trying to arrange peace. He [Owen] is the leader of the Scientologists. They wrote to me recently asking me to stand as their MP in Wales. The SDP lasted for a while and he and Owen bust up, maybe in 1983, after that election. David Steel represents a constituency on the Scottish Border. He was a candidate in the elections in Italy, came fourth out of 16 – I guess he must have made a lot of money from that.

Source: Laws, K. R., McKenna, P. J., & McCarthy, R. A. (1995). Delusions about people. *Neurocase*, 1, 349–362.

Theory of Mind

The concept of theory of mind, the ability to infer the mental states of others, is not something that grew out of observations on patients with brain damage. Instead its origins were in primate psychology and the ideas were later applied to developmental psychology, leading to the spectacularly successful theory that theory of mind impairment is the key cognitive deficit in autism. Only belatedly have circumscribed theory of mind deficits been identified in patients with brain damage, especially those with the frontal lobe syndrome and fronto-temporal dementia (Brüne & Brüne-Cohrs, 2006; Kipps & Hodges, 2006).

How theory of mind abnormality came to be a theory of delusions is due mainly to the work of Frith. In his book, *The Cognitive Neuropsychology of Schizophrenia* (Frith, 1992), he argued that schizophrenic symptoms which involved a feeling of alien control could potentially be understood as a disorder of self-monitoring, specifically a failure to label movements as being self-generated (see Chapter 1). In a similar but more complicated way, he argued that another failure of self-monitoring, this time of inner speech, could give rise to auditory hallucinations. He then made a conceptual leap and suggested that self-monitoring is just one example of a more general failure in the representation of mental states, encompassing both a failure to represent one's own mental states (previously self-monitoring) and now also a failure to represent the mental states of others. Representation of other people's mental states is simply another way of saying theory of mind, and this led Frith to propose that impairment in this ability, arising de novo in adult life, could give rise to both referential and propositional delusions:

> The failure of metarepresentation associated with adult schizophrenia may well be qualitatively different from that associated with childhood autism. The autistic child does not try to infer the mental states of others. In contrast, adult schizophrenic patients, because their early development has been relatively normal, will continue to make inferences about the mental states of others, but will often get these wrong. They will 'see' intentions to communicate when none are there (delusions of reference). They may start to believe that people are deliberately behaving in such a way as to disguise their intentions. They will deduce that there is a general conspiracy against them and that people's intentions towards them are evil (paranoid delusions).

Frith's (1992) proposal set in motion a wave of studies investigating theory of mind in schizophrenia. These quickly established that performance was impaired on tests ranging from adult versions of the classical false belief task used in autistic children (Frith & Corcoran, 1996; Doody et al., 1998), to those examining the ability to understanding implied meaning (Corcoran et al., 1995), or to get jokes that depend on understanding what is in a person's mind (Corcoran et al., 1997). Two meta-analyses (Sprong et al., 2007; Bora et al., 2009) later found that the degree of impairment was substantial and larger than could be attributed to any accompanying general intellectual impairment.

The important question, however, is not whether performance on theory of mind tasks is impaired in schizophrenia, but whether it is related to delusions. On the face of it, the answer would be predicted to be no, since this would violate the principle established above that reality distortion is not associated with any kind of cognitive deficit. And so it proved: while initial studies by Frith and co-workers (Corcoran et al., 1995; Corcoran & Frith, 1996; Frith & Corcoran, 1996; Corcoran et al., 1997) tended to support the view that patients with symptoms such as alien control and persecutory delusions showed poor performance on theory of mind tests, a later meta-analysis of six studies examining the correlations between performance on various theory of mind tests and Liddle's three syndromes (Ventura et al., 2013) revealed the familiar pattern of significant correlations with negative symptoms ($r = -0.25$) and disorganization ($r = -0.32$) but not reality distortion ($r = -0.08$).

One study seems particularly damning in this respect. Walston et al. (2000) conducted a search for patients with psychotic illnesses characterized only by delusions. They were able to find four such cases; none of them showed other schizophrenic symptoms, and they would probably have qualified for a diagnosis of delusional disorder (although the authors did not apply diagnostic criteria). They were all intellectually relatively intact, defined in terms of scores above the cut-off for cognitive impairment on a widely used measure of this (the Mini-Mental State Examination, MMSE). All four patients scored at ceiling or close to this on three theory of mind tests. A summary of one of the patients is shown in Box 5.1, which also makes it clear that he had no difficulty attributing mental states to his imaginary persecutors.

> **Box 5.1** Theory of Mind in a Patient with Delusions and No Other Symptoms (Walston et al., 2000)
>
> Case A was 40-year-old married man who was married with three children. His delusional beliefs started to form the day after he was involved in a fight in which he seriously injured a man. He thought that he was overheard making disparaging remarks about drug dealers whilst at work one day, and that this conversation was reported back to the drug 'mafia' who concluded that he must be a police informer. After this incident, he began to notice that he was being followed by groups of young men who operated from a fleet of cars, both of which changed over time, and he came to believe that they wanted to catch and kill him because they believed he was a 'supergrass'. As a result, he ran away from home and began to live rough, hiding out in remote country areas, and moving frequently from place to place. After some days, however, he became physically and emotionally exhausted, and returned home where he became depressed, consumed large quantities of alcohol, and made a suicide attempt. This led to him being admitted to hospital where he was treated with neuroleptics and antidepressants.
>
> Since his initial stay in hospital, Case A has been readmitted and continues as an outpatient. Three years on, after further in-patient and out-patient care, he was hopeful that the drug mafia may have realized – as a result of their intense surveillance – that they had been targeting an innocent man.
>
> The three theory of mind tests used in the study included two sets of humorous cartoons, one of which involved 'physical' i.e. slapstick humour and the other of which required making inferences concerning mental states to get the joke. The second test involved interpretation of theory of mind narratives, and the third was designed to measure understanding of the meaning of hints. Case A scored 10/10 on the hinting task, 17/17 on the narratives, and 5/5 on each on the physical and theory of mind cartoon tasks. One of the theory of mind cartoons pictured a house with a sign at the front gate saying 'Beware of the bog' instead of the typical 'Beware of the dog'. However, in the garden a man is in fact sinking in a bog. Case's A's explanation was: '"Beware of the bog" and he's laughing because he thinks they've spelt it wrong.'
>
> Analysis of Case A's description of his persecution also revealed that he was able to make sophisticated ToM inferences concerning the mental states of others, specifically his pursuers:
>
> 1. They must think to themselves now they've made right plonkers [idiots] of themselves, mustn't they? I'm not a supergrass…
> 2. When that happened they must have thought, 'it's that swine over there, he's tipped them off, he'll know'.
> 3. They must watch me twenty-four hours a day and think, 'We know he's a police informer, we think we know he is, but by God we've never seen him talk to the Police, or anything like that.'

Of course, the cognitive neuropsychological approach permits and even encourages thinking in terms of abnormalities that are not impairments. Frith (2004) himself acknowledged this in relation to theory of mind:

> It is misleading to refer to the problem as a theory of mind deficit in the case of schizophrenia. A person who does not have a theory of mind takes no account of the beliefs and desires of other people when trying to understand their behaviour. Indeed, he may not have any concept of beliefs and desires. This may be the case in schizophrenic patients with predominantly negative features, but not in those with positive symptoms. The patient with paranoid delusions has no problem ascribing intentions to other people. His problem is that he ascribes the wrong intentions. He has a theory of mind since he explains the behaviour of others in terms of their intentions. The fault lies in the mechanism that is used to discover what these intentions are.

The problem is that very few studies have ventured into such territory. In a small study of 12 patients with persecutory delusions (8 with schizophrenia and 4 with affective disorder) and 10 without persecutory delusions (3 with schizophrenia and 7 with affective disorder), Blakemore et al. (2003) found that the former group tended to read intentions into the movements of two abstract shapes that moved around a screen when there was nothing in the shapes' movements to actually suggest this. In another, larger study (Montag et al., 2011), 80 schizophrenic patients and 80 well-matched controls watched videotaped scenes of social interactions involving false belief, faux pas, metaphor or sarcasm. When asked about what had happened in the scenes, the patients made more errors than the controls, not only on probe questions that referred to a lack of awareness of the characters' intentions, but also on questions where the wrong intentions were attributed to the actors. There was some evidence of an association between these latter 'overmentalizing' responses and delusions, but this was not robust (i.e. it disappeared when potential confounding factors were controlled for).

Into the Realm of Cognitive Psychology

For some aspects of cognitive function, trying to make an explicit link with particular parts of the brain is neither necessary nor desirable. Of course, like everything else these processes depend ultimately on brain function being intact, but they reflect the contribution of many different underlying systems. In the same way as for cognitive neuropsychological approaches but even more so, the concept of malfunction in such systems is freed from the straitjacket of loss of function: it now becomes relatively easy to think in terms of hyperfunction and the novel concept of biased function also begins to make an appearance. Three approaches to delusions stand out as being purely cognitive psychological in this sense. As it happens, they break down quite neatly according to the time period when they arose: the old if not particularly venerable tradition of disordered logic in schizophrenia, followed by Maher's theory of the deluded patient as a naïve scientist, and finally the proposal that delusions are due to probabilistic reasoning bias, or 'jumping to conclusions' as it is popularly known.

Delusions = Disordered Logic

The possibility that delusions might be the result of a problem with logical reasoning was first formally proposed by Von Domarus (1944), in a somewhat whimsical article that seems to have been cited much more frequently than it has actually been read. After an introduction that took in the developmental theories of Vygotsky, the behaviour of an elephant in a zoo that wanted a piece of sugar from a visitor, and the role of mime in mute mentally handicapped patients, he went on to describe two schizophrenic patients who showed a peculiar disturbance of logic. The first believed that the number that 21 meant bathing station. His reasoning went as follows: 21 = 12, 12 means the twelfth month, and the twelfth month is the end of the year; one bathes at the end of the year, and the new year is no longer the old or the reverse of the old year. The second patient considered that Jesus, cigar boxes and sex were identical. Questioning revealed a link involving the idea of being encircled. Thus, the head of Jesus is encircled by a halo, a package of cigars is encircled by a tax band, and a woman 'is encircled by the sex glance of a man'.

Von Domarus (1944) identified these two patients' underlying problem as a failure of Aristotelian syllogistic reasoning. Thus, the syllogism 'All men are mortal; Socrates is a man;

therefore Socrates is mortal' is true. In contrast 'Certain Indians are swift; stags are swift; therefore certain Indians are stags' is false. Some people (including the present author) might find it difficult to put their finger on just what the crucial difference between the two sets of propositions is, but the important point is that if there is a failure of logical reasoning in schizophrenia, delusions could plausibly be the result.

Over the next thirty years or so, chronically hospitalized schizophrenic patients across America found themselves being challenged with the kinds of logical problems shown in Box 5.2. Nearly all the studies (Gottesman & Chapman, 1960; Williams, 1964; Coyle & Bernard, 1965; Ho, 1974) were carried out in the days before there were diagnostic criteria for schizophrenia. Nor was much consideration given to the possible confounding effects of general intellectual impairment on performance, although two of the studies did match the patients and controls for current IQ (Coyle et al., 1965; Watson & Wold, 1981). The results were not very encouraging: three studies found no significant difference from controls (Williams et al., 1964; Coyle et al., 1965; Watson et al., 1981), and in the other two (Gottesman and Chapman, 1960; Ho, 1974) differences were only found on some of the tests used.

Box 5.2 Examples of Logical Problems Used in Studies of Reasoning in Schizophrenia

All Tom's ties are red.
 Some of the things Ada is holding are red.
 Therefore:
1. At least some of the things Ada is holding are Tom's ties.
2. At least some of the things Ada is holding are not Tom's ties.
3. None of these conclusions is proved.
4. None of the things Ada is holding are Tom's ties.
5. All the things Ada is holding are Tom's ties.

(Gottesman and Chapman, 1960)

If some frogs are poetic, and some frogs are bullies, then:
1. All bullies are poetic.
2. Some poetic animals are not bullies.
3. No valid conclusion possible.
4. Some bullies are poetic.
5. Some poetic animals are bullies.

(Williams, 1964)

Two hundred students in their early teens voluntarily attended a recent weekend student conference in a Midwestern city. At this conference, the topics of race relations and means of achieving lasting world peace were discussed, because these were the problems the students selected as being most vital in today's world. For each inference below respond true, probably true, insufficient data, probably false or false.

1. As a group, the students who attended this conference showed a keener interest in broad social problems than do most other students in their early teens.
2. The majority of the students had not previously discussed the conference topics in their schools.

3. The students came from all sections of the country.
4. The students discussed mainly labor relations problems.
5. Some teenage students felt it worthwhile to discuss problems of race relations and ways of achieving world peace.

(Coyle and Bernard, 1965)

If the radio is on, then there is no music.

(a) If the radio is not on, then there is no music.
(b) If the radio is on, then someone must be around.
(c) The radio is on, and there is no music.
(d) If there is music, then the radio is on.
(e) None of the above.

(Ho, 1974)

All dogs are animals. All animals eat. Therefore (choose one):

1. All animals are dogs.
2. All dogs eat.
3. Eating animals are dogs.
4. Only dogs eat.

(Watson et al., 1976)

What none of these studies investigated was whether logical reasoning impairment in schizophrenia was related to delusions. Years later this omission was rectified by Kemp et al. (1997). They examined 16 chronically psychotic patients who showed prominent delusions (according to DSM-III-R criteria 14 had schizophrenia, one had delusional disorder and one had atypical psychosis). They were all of average or above-average estimated premorbid IQ and none showed evidence of generalized intellectual impairment as measured, somewhat crudely, using the MMSE. They and 16 matched controls were given a series of syllogisms and conditional logical problems similar to those in Box 5.2. As in the study of Rossell et al. (1998), some of the problems were also deliberately altered to make them emotional, touching on themes of religion, illness and violence. The authors also added a third form of reasoning test based on Tversky and Kahneman's work on heuristics (see Chapter 4). This involved problems of the following type:

Linda is 31 years old, single, outspoken and very bright. She got a degree in philosophy. As a student she was deeply concerned with issues of discrimination and social justice, and also participated in antinuclear demonstrations. Linda:-

(a) is a bank clerk and is active in the feminist movement.
(b) is a plumber.
(c) is a bank clerk.

The correct answer is (c). Many people choose (a) although it is wrong, because by definition there are more women who are bank clerks than who are bank clerks and active in the feminist movement – the so-called conjunction fallacy. This test is notorious for its ability to induce incorrect responding, even among intelligent and sophisticated people (it is said, possibly apocryphally, that statisticians perform especially poorly on it).

The patients and controls were found to perform equally well on the syllogisms and conditionals, or rather equally badly since they both endorsed high numbers of wrong answers. There were some, although not very clear, suggestions of a pattern of worse performance by the patients on the emotional problems. In contrast, the deluded patients actually performed slightly better than the controls on the problems involving heuristics, in the sense of not being misled by the normal tendency to opt for the conjunction fallacy. Overall, the authors concluded that differences in reasoning between deluded patients and controls were surprisingly small.

The Deluded Patient as Naïve Scientist

In retrospect, the disordered logic theory never had much hope of being successful, for the simple reason that it essentially proposed that delusions were related to a cognitive deficit, albeit a rather esoteric one. This trap was avoided in the next historically important approach, which actually made a virtue out of intactness in a cognitive system. This was Maher's (1974; Maher & Ross, 1984) proposal that delusions arise when processes fundamentally indistinguishable from those used by normal individuals to explain novel events are brought to bear on the abnormal perceptual experiences that occur in schizophrenia.

According to the theory, the process of delusion formation begins when a patient in the early stages of schizophrenia finds him- or herself having strange experiences. These experiences appear important, partly because they are new and mysterious, and partly because of the fact that they are often overwhelmingly intense. They demand an explanation, and this is achieved by a process of data collection and hypothesis testing which is similar in all important respects to the methods used in science. The process typically takes place in the following stages:

1. Initial observation: Unexpected or anomalous events create a feeling of significance in the observer that requires explanation.
2. Experience of puzzlement: The individual experiences a state describable as puzzled, curious, confused and surprised. This leads to first checking that the observation is actually what it seems to be and not something else, and secondly a search for other events that might be related to it. During this stage the individual begins to develop a tentative hypothesis about the event.
3. Additional observations: The state of puzzlement prompts a search for additional data. This may support the initial hypothesis, but if not it is rejected or amended, and the process is repeated until one hypothesis begins to gain ground.
4. The explanatory insight: Sooner or later the individual arrives at a point where the mystery seems to be solved – a kind of eureka moment where everything suddenly becomes clear. This has an emotional component, which may be marked (Maher and Ross (1984) quoted a biochemist who described the moment of scientific discovery as 'a pure and primitive happiness deeper than anything of this kind which can ever be granted to a human being to experience').
5. The process of confirmation: An explanation has now been arrived at, but its adequacy still needs to be tested. Although this might be expected to be an objective process, the reality is that once a firm conclusion has been reached it is likely to be held on to tenaciously in

the way that normal beliefs tend to be, as described in Chapter 4. Another factor might be the belief's quasi-scientific nature; Maher and Ross (1984) noted how important scientific discoveries are often rejected by the discoverer's contempories before ultimately being hailed as works of genius.

The end result would be a propositional delusion. According to Maher (1974), the content of this – religious, political or quasi-scientific – would reflect the patient's particular cultural background. Persecutory delusions might additionally arise as a result of the patients finding that other people do not seem to share their experiences, leading them to conclude that they are being lied to. Or they might decide that they are extraordinary because they have been selected to have experiences denied to others. Events in the patients' own history could also play a part: a person who had a guilty secret might conclude that he or she was being punished for this.

For Maher the abnormal experiences that the patient needed to explain were principally a range of perceptual anomalies that occurred in the early stages of schizophrenia. He cited the case of Schreber, a judge who wrote about his own psychotic illness (in a book that later formed the basis of Freud's psychoanalytic explanation of delusions): his initial symptoms were bodily sensations which ultimately led him to conclude that he was changing into a woman. In other cases it could be pains or the smelling of unpleasant odours. Maher also placed considerable emphasis on an alleged heightening of perception in the early stages of schizophrenia that had been described in a paper by McGhie and Chapman (1961).

An obvious difficulty for the naïve scientist theory is what happens when there no perceptual abnormalities of any kind, as can sometimes be the case in schizophrenia (and is the rule in delusional disorder). Maher and Ross (1984) got round this problem by proposing that in these circumstances there was a 'central neuropathology', which caused normal experiences to be imbued with a feeling of special significance; he explicitly identified the resulting state as delusional mood. The same hypothesis testing machinery could then be brought into play to produce an explanation for this experience.

Even with this patch, Maher's theory faced problems. One was that it predicted that patients with full-blown hallucinations would always develop delusional explanations of them, something that is by no means always the case. It also predicted that non-psychotic individuals with conditions such as tinnitus and the phantom limb syndrome ought to develop delusions based on these experiences. Nothing of the kind has ever been described so far as the present author knows. Finally, it failed to explain why schizophrenic delusions tend to be bizarre or fantastic – an essentially normal hypothesis-testing process should produce explanations that incline to the mundane and plausible.

None of these problems is necessarily insurmountable, and it is possible that more sophisticated versions of Maher's proposal could have found ways to deal with them. However, no such revised theory has ever been presented, something that probably reflects the fact that even the simple form of the theory has never been subjected to any kind of empirical testing. This does not mean, however, that it has not been influential. For example, it features in the integrative model of delusions proposed by a group of contemporary British researchers (Garety et al., 2001; Freeman et al., 2002; Freeman, 2007). Maher's suggestions as to how propositional delusions can form out of abnormal significance and be coloured by the patient's culture and life experiences also crop up again in the salience theory of delusions discussed in Chapter 8.

Probabilistic Reasoning Bias

The origins of the third cognitive approach to delusions go back to a theoretical paper by Hemsley and Garety (1986) in which they considered the question of whether delusions could be understood as an alteration in the way in people normally reach conclusions based on the balance of probabilities. Their argument was inspired by a mathematical treatment of such hypothetical processes using the principles of Bayesian inference (Fischhoff & Beyth-Marom, 1983). They were also impressed by a study of patients with obsessive-compulsive disorder, which had found that they required more evidence than healthy controls to reach a decision in a task requiring judgement under uncertainty (Volans, 1976). It seemed at least possible that patients with delusions might require less evidence than normal to do so.

Two years later Hemsley, Garety and co-workers published the results of a study designed to answer this question (Huq et al., 1988). Fifteen schizophrenic patients with delusions, 10 patients with other psychiatric diagnoses and 15 healthy controls were shown two jars, one of which, the experimenter explained, contained 85 beads of one colour and 15 beads of a different colour, and the other of which contained beads in the reverse proportions. The containers were then hidden from view and the subjects were informed that beads would be drawn from one jar only, replaced, the jar shaken, another bead drawn, and so on, until they felt confident they knew which jar the beads were being taken from. (In fact, unknown to the subjects, the beads were always drawn in the same pre-arranged sequence that favoured a decision after several draws). The experimental design is summarized in Figure 5.2. As predicted, the schizophrenic patients were found to require significantly less draws to decision than both the healthy subjects and the psychiatric controls. Some of them reached a decision after only seeing one bead.

Eleven years later, Garety and Freeman (1999) reviewed this and seven more studies that had since been carried out. These studies all used the beads task, although sometimes in proportions such as 60:40 or 75:25, and one study also employed additional versions of the task designed to be either more realistic (deciding whether children's names were from a 'mainly boys' or 'mainly girls' category) or more emotionally salient (deciding whether comments about people were from a 'mainly positive' or 'mainly negative' survey). All but one of the studies replicated the finding of 'jumping to conclusions' in schizophrenic patients. One study also found the effect in patients with delusional disorder.

Another ten years or so later, the same authors (Garety & Freeman, 2013) reviewed the literature again, by which time the number of studies had ballooned to nearly 70. Many studies continued to use beads, but by now there were a number of paradigms involving two kinds of fish, or words with both neutral and emotional content. The ratio of positive to negative findings was less favourable than in their earlier review, but the authors still found that a clear majority of studies found evidence for jumping to conclusions, with on average about half of patients with schizophrenia coming to a confident decision in two draws or less.

By this time, and bearing in mind the experience with theory of mind, the question on everyone's lips was whether jumping to conclusions was a function of being deluded, or just of having schizophrenia. Garety and Freeman (2013) felt that there was every reason to believe that the former was the case, pointing out that the larger studies usually found evidence of an association with delusions. The study they singled out in this respect, however, was less than reassuring: Lincoln et al. (2010) examined 71 psychotic patients and found that draws to decision was not significantly correlated with any clinical variable in the easy 80:20 condition. There was a significant correlation with delusion scores in the harder 60:40 condition;

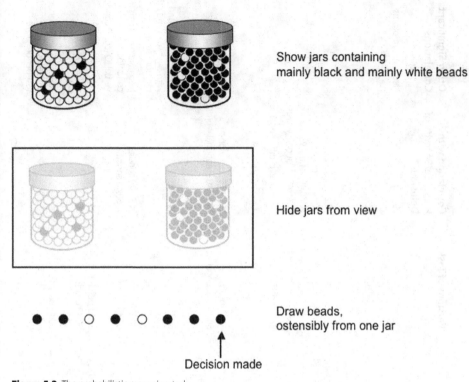

Show jars containing
mainly black and mainly white beads

Hide jars from view

Draw beads,
ostensibly from one jar

Decision made

Figure 5.2 The probabilistic reasoning task.

however, when either negative symptoms or current IQ, which were also correlated with draws to decision, were controlled for in the analysis, the result became non-significant.

This and other studies examining the relationship between jumping to conclusions and delusions are shown in Table 5.3. Some of them compared matched groups of patients with and without delusions, whereas others took a correlational approach, or used multiple regression analysis which has the advantage of being able to remove the potential confounding effects of other variables also associated with delusions and/or draws to decision. It is clear that their findings are not nearly as supportive as Garety and Freeman (2013) would like to believe. Most studies found no significant relationship with delusions. One study found a trend-level association and in two others there was a significant association in only one of the conditions used. A meta-analysis of these and a few other studies (e.g. imaging studies) from which data could be extracted (Dudley et al., 2016) also found the pooled correlation between draws to decision and delusion scores to be insignificant at -0.09.

What Table 5.3 does reveal are hints that jumping to conclusions is associated with negative symptoms and poor performance on neuropsychological tests. The latter finding, in particular, raises the possibility that probabilistic reasoning bias may not be a bias at all, but instead a cognitive deficit. Further support for this interpretation comes from a study by Lunt et al. (2012), which gave the beads task to 19 neurological patients with frontal lobe lesions. The patients were found to show significantly reduced draws to decision compared

Table 5.3 Studies Examining the Relationship of Jumping to Conclusions to Delusions

Study	Sample	Diagnoses	Analysis	Versions of Task	Correlation with Presence/Severity of Delusions?	Other Significant Correlations
Mortimer et al. (1996)	43	Schizophrenia	Simple correlation	85:15	✗	Negative symptoms
Moritz & Woodward (2005)	31	Schizophrenia	Compared age and sex matched subgroups with and without delusions	90:10 beads	✗	-
Menon et al. (2006)	33	Schizophrenia	Compared age, sex and premorbid IQ matched subgroups with and without delusions	85:15 beads 60:40 beads 60:40 neutral words 60:40 emotional words	✗ 85:15 condition ✗ 60:40 condition ✗ 60:40 neutral words ✗ 60:40 emotional words	-
Peters et al. (2008)	37	Schizophrenia, schizo-affective disorder, psychosis NOS, bipolar disorder	Compared age and sex matched subgroups with high and low delusion scores	85:15 beads	? (trend level difference)	-
Colbert et al. (2010)	34	First or second episode psychosis excluding organic diagnoses and bipolar disorder	Compared numbers meeting criterion for JTC bias in groups with and without current delusions	85:15 beads 60:40 emotional words	✗ 85:15 condition ✗ 60:40 emotional words	-
Langdon et al. (2010)	35	Schizophrenia, schizo-affective disorder	Simple correlation	85:15 beads	✗	No correlation found with digit span and other memory scores
Lincoln et al. (2010)	71	Nonaffective psychosis	Simple correlation	80:20 beads 60:40 beads	✗ 80:20 condition ✓ 60:40 condition	Negative symptoms (60:40 condition) Verbal IQ (60:40 condition)
Dudley et al. (2011)	77	First-episode psychosis patients, not further specified	Compared age and sex matched subgroups with and without delusions	85:15 beads 60:40 beads	✗ ✗	-
Buck et al. (2012)	40	Schizophrenia, schizo-affective disorder	Simple correlation	60:40 beads	✗	No significant association with executive or memory test performance

Study	N	Diagnosis	Analysis	Conditions	Association with JTC	Other measures
So et al. (2012)*	273	Schizophrenia, schizo-affective disorder, delusional disorder	Simple correlation	85:15 beads, 60:40 beads, 60:40 emotional words	✗ 85:15 condition, ✗ 60:40 condition, ✗ emotional words	Negative symptoms, Current IQ, Digit span, Working memory
Freeman et al. (2014)	123	Non-affective psychosis	Logistic regression	60:40 beads	✗ 60:40 condition	-
Ochoa et al. (2014)	43	Schizophrenia	Logistic regression	85:15 beads, 60:40 beads, 60:40 emotional words	✗ 85:15 condition, ✗ 60:40 condition, ✗ emotional words	Significant associations with 2 out of 14 neuropsychological measures, not consistent across beads/words conditions
Falcone et al. (2015)	108	First-episode psychosis, one-third with affective diagnoses	Logistic regression	85:15 beads, 60:40 beads	✓ 85:15 condition, ✗ 60:40 condition	Current IQ, Spatial working memory

*Includes patients from study of Garety et al. (2013)

to 25 healthy controls, and this was associated with poor performance on some but not all of a range of measures of executive functioning also administered as part of the study.

Conclusion: Can Anything Be Salvaged from the Wreckage?

In many ways, a psychological theory of delusions seems as far away as it must have done half a century ago when the first tentative steps in this direction were being taken. The theories themselves are not particularly powerful: only one of them has had anything to say about referential delusions and none of them provide an explanation of why propositional delusions show the typical features of being fixed, incorrigible, bizarre or even fantastic. None of the theories have emerged unscathed from empirical testing, and several of them, it has to be said, have not stood up to it very well at all.

One avenue that seems closed forever is the idea of delusions being due to a cognitive deficit. This applies not just to neuropsychological deficits – including the perennial favourite of schizophrenia research, executive function – but also it seems to any other kind of cognitive disturbance that can be conceptualized in such a way. If such a deficit did exist it would have to be one that (a) is currently unknown and (b) is spared by the general tendency to intellectual impairment that also characterizes schizophrenia. What makes this conclusion especially harsh is that it brings down with it an ingenious and much-loved theoretical approach to delusions, theory of mind impairment. Probabilistic reasoning bias may be another casualty here: its association with neuropsychological test impairment in schizophrenia and the fact that it is also seen in patients with frontal lobe lesions make it look suspiciously like a deficit in disguise.

Cognitive neuropsychiatry offers a potential way out of this impasse. Semantic memory is a plausible place to look for a non-deficit abnormality, if for no other reason than the fact that delusions seem to reside in one particular subdivision of this, personal semantic memory. Nevertheless, in terms of experimental support, the semantic memory theory of delusions hangs by the slenderest of threads – faint signals of altered factual knowledge in areas related to delusions in Rossell et al.'s (1998) study, and suggestions of something not too dissimilar from the single case study of Laws et al. (1995). Even if semantic memory is affected, there is no real idea of what form the disturbance might take – disorganization of the network architecture? an excessive tendency to lay down semantic memories? – all possibilities seem to lie deep in the realm of speculation. An 'overmentalizing' form of theory of mind dysfunction could also work, but the same theoretical reservations apply, and the almost complete lack of studies investigating this possibility does not inspire confidence.

Maher's theory remains untested. Patients with schizophrenia have no more problems with logical reasoning than anyone else, and the hints from Kemp et al.'s (1997) study that something more than this is going on are if anything slighter than in the case of semantic memory. Probabilistic reasoning bias is not convincingly associated with presence of delusions. The only remaining candidate for a psychological theory of delusions is the third cognitive neuropsychological approach alluded to at the beginning of the chapter, whose starting point is the occurrence of delusion-like phenomena in neurological disease. Whether this approach can succeed where others have failed, and whether it can get round the problem that deficits are not associated with delusions in psychiatric disorders, is examined in Chapter 7. But before doing so a whole different approach to delusions needs to be considered.

The Neurochemical Connection

As psychology struggled to make headway with delusions, another discipline close to the heart of psychiatry, pharmacology, was sending out signals that a different approach might be more successful. The psychopharmacological era began in 1952 with the discovery that a drug, chlorpromazine, brought about substantial clinical benefit in schizophrenia, where everything everything else from psychoanalysis to insulin coma therapy had previously failed. Not only did this and other antipsychotic drugs improve psychotic symptoms, it seemed that other drugs could also induce them in healthy people. This became clear a few years later when psychiatry finally accepted what had been staring it in the face for years, that amphetamine not-infrequently produced a state indistinguishable from schizophrenia in people who used it.

Antipsychotic drugs exert their therapeutic effects by producing a functional decrease in brain dopamine; amphetamine and other stimulants cause a functional increase of the same neurotransmitter. These two complementary findings became the pillars of the dopamine hypothesis of schizophrenia, which reigned supreme for a quarter of a century, until a competitor arrived in the form of a drug with effects on another neurotransmitter. Phencyclidine, which had been introduced in the 1950s, was known to induce vivid subjective experiences in many patients who were given it as an anaesthetic or for pre-operative sedation, and it had even been investigated as a possible pharmacological model for schizophrenia. Later it became a drug of abuse and users started to turn up in emergency rooms in severe psychotic states. Later still it was found to act by blocking the N-methyl-D-aspartate (NMDA) receptor, one of several classes of glutamate receptor.

The dopamine hypothesis survives to the present day despite a number of reversals of fortune. At the time of writing, the glutamate theory is facing an existential crisis, due mainly to the failure of any of a range of glutamatergic drugs to show therapeutic effectiveness in schizophrenia. But this is beside the point; all that matters for present purposes is that disturbances in one or both of these neurotransmitters can cause healthy people to experience delusions. On this basis, another neurotransmitter system, the endocannabinoid system, also needs to be considered. Although not in the same league as dopamine and glutamate as a neurochemical theory of schizophrenia, cannabis certainly punches above its weight in terms of its ability to induce psychotic symptoms in healthy people.

Dopamine

Stimulant Drug-Induced Psychosis

The apparent ability of amphetamine to induce delusions and other psychotic symptoms was first noted in 1938, in three patients who had started taking the drug for narcolepsy (Young & Scoville, 1938). Hundreds of further case reports followed, which also implicated other stimulant drugs such as phenmetrazine and methylphenidate, and even some over the counter preparations such as ephedrine and diethylpropion (Angrist & Sudilovsky, 1978). Stimulant drug users themselves recognized the problem of 'speed paranoia' (Rylander 1972; Schiorring 1981). However, it was only after Connell (1958) published a detailed analysis of 42 cases of amphetamine psychosis that resistance to the idea of a causal link finally evaporated. He demolished the argument that what was being seen was a toxic-confusional state. His case material also provided little support for an alternative argument that amphetamine psychosis was simply schizophrenia being 'released' in predisposed individuals who had drifted into drug use as part of their evolving illness.

Nevertheless, stimulant drug-induced psychosis is a less than ideal neurochemical model for delusions. One reason why is the fact that it induces other psychotic symptoms as well. Thus, several of Connell's (1958) patients had auditory and other hallucinations, and formal thought disorder was also evident in some of the cases he described in detail. Subsequent studies have made it clear that the entire clinical picture of schizophrenia can be reproduced, including negative symptoms and catatonic phenomena up to and including stupor (Tatetsu, 1964; Chen et al., 2003). Nevertheless, there is probably some truth to the widely quoted view that stimulant-induced psychosis tends to take the form of a paranoid-hallucinatory state. For example, in their series of 174 methamphetamine users with psychosis in Taiwan, Chen et al. (2003) found that delusions were present in 71 per cent and hallucinations in 84 per cent, but only around 5 per cent showed disorganized speech (although a further 27 per cent were described as having speech that was odd).

Another problem for the model is that the immediate effects of stimulant drugs are euphoria and increased alertness; psychosis is something that occurs later and then not in everyone. How much later and with what frequency has never been satisfactorily established. Thirty of Connell's 42 cases were using amphetamine regularly, but 8 developed psychosis after taking a single large dose of the drug. In Chen et al.'s (2003) study of methamphetamine users, less than half had ever experienced psychotic symptoms, despite the fact that they were prisoners on remand for drug-related offences, and so their use was presumably extensive. (This is also the present author's experience: he and a colleague once administered the lifetime version of the PSE to around 30 regular stimulant drug users. Although some gave clear retrospective descriptions of psychotic symptoms, it was striking how many had never experienced anything more than vague concerns that the police might be watching them, despite taking the drug in positively veterinary doses.) In an experimental study, Griffith et al. (1968) administered hourly doses of amphetamine to four abstinent users and found that they all developed paranoid and referential delusions within a few days. However, in another study of the same type (Angrist & Gershon, 1970), only two out of four subjects developed clear-cut psychotic states, with the other two showing only at most questionable symptoms, for example becoming hostile and suspicious, or hearing their names being called.

Virtually all the evidence points to the psychosis-inducing effects of stimulants being due to an effect on dopamine. As a group, these drugs act to increase the synaptic release of the monoamine neurotransmitters dopamine and noradrenalin, which is achieved by a variety of mechanisms (Iversen, 2008a). However, most if not all of the effects in animals appear to be due to an action on the former transmitter; it is difficult to provoke any behavioural change at all by pharmacological manipulation of noradrenalin (Mason, 1984). Likewise, in man, psychotic symptoms are a well-documented side effect of l-DOPA and other dopamine agonist drugs used in Parkinson's disease (Cummings, 1991). In contrast, despite occasional claims to the contrary (Yamamoto & Hornykiewicz, 2004), psychosis is not a recognized complication of treatment with tricyclic antidepressants, which block re-uptake of noradrenalin, nor any of a range of other drugs with noradrenergic actions.

Many stimulant drugs also lead to increased synaptic release of a third monoamine neurotransmitter, serotonin. This also seems to be a red herring, however, since methylphenidate (Ritalin) is well documented as causing psychotic symptoms in children with attention deficit-hyperactivity disorder, (Lucas & Weiss, 1971; Mosholder et al., 2009), even though it has minimal effects on serotonin neurons (Kuczenski & Segal, 1997; see also Iversen, 2008a).

What Does Dopamine Do in the Brain?

Of a small number of central nervous system pathways that use dopamine, the only one relevant to behaviour is the so-called mesotelencephalic dopamine system. As described by Bjorklund and Dunnett (2007) in the most recent summary of their and others' 30 plus years work in the field, this pathway arises from a group of cells in the midbrain, including A9 in the substantia nigra bilaterally and A10 in the midline ventral tegmental area between them; there are also two A8 groups lying behind A9 in the retrorubral area. In the past, much has been made of the separation of A9 and A10, but the reality is that the whole group of cells forms a continuous sheet. If there is a meaningful anatomical division, it is between a dorsal tier (containing cells from all three groups) and a ventral tier (containing representatives only of A9 and A10).

The total number of dopamine neurons in A8, A9 and A10 is small: 40,000–45,000 in rats, 160,000–320,000 in monkeys and 400,000–600,000 in humans (Bjorklund & Dunnett, 2007). However, the area they innervate is wide: it includes importantly the basal ganglia, specifically the caudate nucleus and putamen (jointly referred to as the striatum), and the ventral extension of these nuclei to two small adjacent structures, the nucleus accumbens and olfactory tubercle (the ventral sectors of the caudate and putamen plus these two nuclei are termed the ventral striatum). Mesotelencephalic dopamine neurons also reach the amygdala, the hippocampus and other limbic structures. In rats, the cortical distribution of dopamine is largely confined to the entorhinal cortex and parts of the cingulate cortex. In monkeys it is more extensive, and in man the entire cortex receives dopamine input. Dorsal regions of the striatum receive their innervation from A9 and the ventral striatum from A10. All non-striatal regions receive dopamine input from A8, A9 and A10.

It has been recognized for a long time that mesotelencephalic dopamine neurons have unusually large and dense terminal arborizations. A recent study by Matsuda et al. (2009), which applied a novel tracing technique to eight nigrostriatal neurons in the rat, found this to be even greater than previously thought, with the region covered by each axonal bush ranging from 0.5 per cent to nearly 6 per cent of the combined volume of the caudate nucleus and putamen. As shown in Figure 6.1, the pattern of arborisation, rather than showing the usual branching tree-like structure, resembles nothing so much as a ball of string.

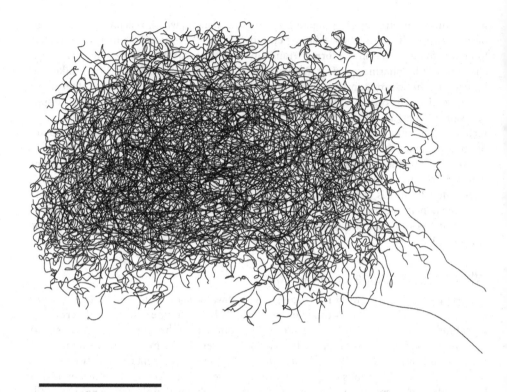

0.5 mm

Figure 6.1 The axonal arborization of a single dopaminergic neuron in the neostriatum, as visualized using a novel viral vector. The axon is on the right and has just divided into two.
Source: Reproduced with permission from Matsuda, W., et al. (2009). Single nigrostriatal dopaminergic neurons form widely spread and highly dense axonal arborizations in the neostriatum. *Journal of Neuroscience, 29*, 444–453.

Because of these anatomical features, it has been long suspected that dopamine exercises some function distinct from conventional neurotransmission. Early conceptualizations of this were in terms of the somewhat vague concept of 'neuromodulation' (e.g. Hornykiewicz, 1976; Bjorklund & Lindvall, 1984; Bloom, 1984). More recently, Agnati and co-workers (Agnati et al., 1986; Zoli & Agnati, 1996; Fuxe et al., 2010) have argued that the mesotelen-cephalic dopamine system is one of several examples of 'volume neurotransmission' in the brain. Here, a neurotransmitter is released, in many cases extrasynaptically as well as intrasynaptically, into the extracellular space bathing other neurons, and exerts diffuse and relatively long-lasting effects on the 'wiring' neurons in the area. In the words of Fuxe et al. (2010):

> The evidence suggests that the main mode of communication of all the three central monoamine neurons ... is short distance (mainly in the mm range) volume [VT] transmission. In many regions their combined existence as diffusing VT signals in the extracellular fluid in concentrations that vary with their pattern of release will have a major impact on the modulation of the polymorphic wiring networks in the CNS. In this way it becomes possible to understand how the [dopamine, noradrenalin and serotonin] terminal networks can have such a powerful role in CNS functions

such as mood, reward, fear, cognition, attention, arousal, motor function, neuroendocrine function and autonomic function and indeed play a central role in neuropsychopharmacology.

What this role translates into in the case of dopamine is the subject of two proposals that are both compelling, but which are not easy to reconcile with one another. The first is that dopamine exerts some facilitatory or permissive function over voluntary movement. The main evidence supporting this view is so well known it hardly needs to be spelt out: reduced dopamine causes Parkinson's disease, where it seems to be particularly implicated in the akinesia and bradykinesia of the disorder rather than symptoms such as tremor (e.g. Rodriguez-Oroz et al., 2009; Helmich et al., 2012). Administration of dopamine blocking drugs to animals has analogous effects, and in high doses induces a state of profound immobility known as catalepsy, where the animal, although not paralysed, will remain in an uncomfortable position for minutes at a time (Joyce, 1983; Mason, 1984). In contrast, dopamine agonist drugs such as amphetamine or apomorphine produce a state of hyperactivity which shows the unusual feature that it progressively gives way to stereotypy: rats, for example, engage in an ever-smaller set of behaviours until they end up repetitively performing one or a few responses like sniffing and rearing.

Beyond this, the precise nature of dopamine's role in voluntary movement remains unclear. Theories of basal ganglia function (e.g. Graybiel, 2005; Seger, 2006) usually revolve around these structures being involved in the automatic selection and elaboration of sequences of motor responses. However, the theories are typically silent on what part dopamine plays in this process. For example, in what is perhaps the most celebrated theoretical paper on basal ganglia function in recent years, Alexander and De Long's (1986) concept of a series of parallel cortico–cortical circuits that pass through their dorsal, ventral and other sectors, dopamine is only mentioned in passing, just before the concluding remarks.

Other approaches emphasize the role of the basal ganglia in motor learning, something that draws heavily on the evidence discussed in the next section (Robbins & Everitt, 1992; Yin & Knowlton, 2006). Such theories, however, fail to explain why dopamine should also have a permissive effect on the production of previously learnt motor acts.

There are no such uncertainties in the second theory of the function of the mesotelencephalic dopamine system. This maintains that dopamine is the neural substrate of reward, or more precisely the motivational effects of this and/or its ability to reinforce responses in learning. This theory dates back to Olds and Milner's (1954) discovery of the rewarding properties of electrical brain stimulation. This was followed by experiments which established first that catecholamines were involved in the effect (see Wise, 1978), and later that dopamine rather than noradrenalin was the important neurotransmitter (see Mason, 1984). After something of a lull, during which researchers mainly occupied themselves with trying to show that dopamine also mediated the effects of natural rewards such as food, the pace abruptly changed. Using single cell recording in awake monkeys while they learned a behavioural task, Schultz (1998) was able to show that 75–80 per cent of mesotelencephalic dopamine neurons switched from their usual pattern of tonic activity to phasic bursts when the animal received a reward, for example touching a morsel of food, or receiving a drop of fruit juice. Crucially, when a reward-signalling stimulus such as a light or a tone was introduced into the experimental environment, the phasic activity to the reward would progressively decrease and be replaced by phasic activity to the stimulus. Ultimately, activity in response to the reward itself would cease to occur, although it could be reinstated if the reward was delivered unexpectedly. This pattern of responding characterized A10 dopamine neurons in the ventral tegmental area, and somewhat less frequently A9 neurons in the substantia nigra.

What made these findings so exciting was that they seemed to be obeying the rules of a mathematical model of reward-based learning originally proposed by Bush and Mosteller (1951a,b) and refined by Rescorla and Wagner (1972) (see Glimcher, 2011). According to this model, the reinforcing value that a stimulus which has been paired with reward acquires (i.e. via classical or Pavlovian conditioning) does not simply depend on how many times it has occurred just before the reward, but instead takes into account the degree to which the reward is unexpected. More precisely, it is a function of the difference between the amount of reward experienced on the current trial and a composite of the rewards received on preceding trials – the so-called reward prediction error. Accordingly, when an animal first encounters, say, a large amount of food in a particular environment, being unexpected this generates a large positive reward prediction error which causes learning to start to take place. As the animal repeats the same experience, there comes a point where there will be no difference between the reward that is predicted and the reward that is actually received, and so no further learning occurs or needs to occur. If the reward then for some reason stops being provided, a negative reward prediction error starts to be generated, and what was previously learnt begins to be unlearnt.

Although the idea that mesotelencephalic dopamine codes for reward prediction error is rightly regarded as groundbreaking, it is not without its problems. One leading researcher in the field, Berridge (Berridge & Robinson, 1998; Berridge, 2007), has argued that, rather than providing a learning signal, dopamine only mediates the way in which stimuli associated with reward acquire energizing or motivational effects on behaviour. Somewhat relatedly, Glimcher (2011) has pointed out that it is not easy to see how midbrain dopamine neurons can generate a reward prediction error signal – none of the known afferent inputs to the ventral tegmental area and substantia nigra appear to be capable of providing the information necessary for such a calculation to be performed. But something else is the real elephant in the room: if dopamine codes for reward prediction error, why do patients with Parkinson's disease not show problems with learning alongside the ones they have with voluntary movement? The vast majority of patients with the disorder remain perfectly able to acquire new information, and the existence of even subtle impairments in motor learning has not proved easy to demonstrate experimentally (e.g. Ruitenberg et al., 2015).

Glutamate

The Psychosis-Inducing Effects of NMDA Antagonists

In 1991, Javitt and Zukin published a review article that went on to become the second most highly cited research paper on schizophrenia of the decade. In this, they argued that phencylidine provided a better neurochemical model of schizophrenia than stimulant drugs, because it induced not only delusions and hallucinations but also formal thought disorder, negative symptoms and other symptoms of the disorder as well. When used as a general anaesthetic, they noted, it induced a state reminiscent of catatonic stupor, with the patient becoming unresponsive with open staring eyes, lack of all facial expression and sometimes waxy flexibility. Psychological reactions were also seen when the patients came round, or alternatively when the drug was given for pre-operative sedation. As described in one of the studies Javitt and Zukin (1991) cited (Johnstone et al., 1959), some patients would become restless and agitated, whereas others would be euphoric and sing, recite poetry or whisper words like 'heavenly', 'beautiful' and 'lovely'. One patient stated that he had become a grub and another was convinced he had been shot into space in a sputnik.

These observations led to studies where volunteers were given sub-anaesthetic doses of phencyclidine. This resulted in what Javitt and Zukin (1991) described as a withdrawn, autistic or negativistic state, which in some cases was accompanied by repetitive movements such as rocking, head rolling and grimacing. Many of the subjects also described bizarre perceptual changes: one (Luby et al., 1959) stated that his arm felt like a 20-mile pole with a pin at the end; and another (Davies & Beech, 1960) reported: 'I felt like a flat worm – my head felt solid but below that I felt flat – like a huge skin rug – though if I looked at myself I saw in three dimensions.' Some subjects were also said to develop marked thought disorder with word salad and neologisms (Luby et al., 1959), although examples were not given.

Javitt and Zukin (1991) then went on to describe how schizophrenia-like states were encountered when phencyclidine became a drug of abuse with the street name of angel dust. As its use spread, users began to turn up in emergency rooms across America (and later Britain and Europe) showing agitation, excitement, hallucinations, delusions, paranoia and incoherent speech. These states were often accompanied by confusion, but Javitt and Zukin (1991) pointed out that the psychotic symptoms could persist for days or weeks after the confusion had cleared. Another presentation was of catatonia or the 'frozen addict' syndrome: McCarron et al. (1981) described patients who were motionless and stiff, with their eyes open and staring blankly and their arms or head in bizarre positions. Many were mute and some repeated a word or phrase continuously.

The final piece of the jigsaw was pharmacological. Javitt and Zukin (1991) cited studies which by the beginning of 1990s had demonstrated conclusively that the main action of phencyclidine was to block one particular class of post-synaptic glutamate receptor, the NMDA receptor. The glutamate hypothesis of schizophrenia, the proposal that abnormal glutamatergic function – this time a deficiency rather than an excess – caused the symptoms of the disorder, was born.

Javitt and Zukin's (1991) article unleashed a massive research initiative in schizophrenia, which has so far lasted 25 years but whose results have been mostly disappointing. The majority of studies examining NMDA receptors in post-mortem schizophrenic brain have found no change in numbers compared to controls; a few found decreases in some areas, but these were matched by others which found increases (Hu et al., 2015; Catts et al., 2016). The findings have also been inconsistent for other classes of glutamate receptor (Hu et al., 2015). Nor have there been any convincing findings of alterations in brain glutamate levels in schizophrenia (see McKenna, 2007).

The news is as bad if not worse for attempts to demonstrate that glutamate agonist drugs can improve the symptoms of schizophrenia. Direct glutamate agonists are mostly too rapidly metabolized to be useful, and also have the potential to cause neuronal damage through excitotoxicity. Studies using indirect NMDA agonists such as D-serine and D-cycloserine were meta-analysed by Tuominen et al. (2005); evidence of effectiveness was only found for negative symptoms. These drugs then proved to be devoid of all therapeutic effects in a large well-controlled trial (Buchanan et al., 2007). Finally there was the saga of LY2140023 (also known as pomaglutamed methionil), a direct agonist at glutamatergic presynaptic autoreceptors. This was found to be almost as effective as olanzapine in an initial double-blind, placebo controlled trial (Patil et al., 2007). However, a second trial showed a marked placebo response, which neither LY2140023 nor olanzapine, which was employed as a comparator, separated from (Kinon et al., 2011). Lilly, the company that developed the drug, subsequently announced that a third trial had shown no superiority against placebo and halted further development.

The only element of the glutamate hypothesis that survives is the ability of NMDA receptor antagonists to induce schizophrenia-like symptoms. Krystal et al. (1994) gave an intravenous dose of the phencyclidine-like anaesthetic drug, ketamine (by then phencyclidine had been withdrawn from use after it was found to have neurotoxic effects in animals) or placebo to 19 healthy subjects under double-blind conditions. The subjects experienced alterations in perception similar to those described with phencyclidine: one subject felt like his legs were floating in the air when he was resting on a bed, and another perceived music quietly playing next door as loud. Formal thought disorder was reported to be present in some subjects, although as in previous studies of phencyclidine, no speech samples were provided to support this. Several subjects were described as developing ideas of reference and paranoid thought content, for example thinking that staff in a neighbouring room were talking about them.

Several further studies documented that volunteers given ketamine showed increases in scores on positive symptom scales, and also in some cases negative symptom scales (Adler et al., 1998, 1999; Bowdle et al., 1998; Newcomer et al., 1999; Lahti et al., 2001). However, beyond noting in passing the occurrence of heightened and distorted perception, ideas of reference and, at high dosage, formal thought disorder, these studies did not actually describe the symptoms the subjects experienced. Only one study to date has attempted to do this: Pomarol-Clotet et al. (2006) gave intravenous ketamine or placebo to 15 healthy subjects under double-blind conditions and rated the symptoms they developed using a shortened form of the PSE. Most reported feelings of unreality and changed perception of time, and several described heightening, dulling and distortion of perception. Sometimes these latter changes were quite dramatic: one subject described the interviewer, who was heavily pregnant at the time, gradually coming to look like a dome with a pair of eyes on top. However, as in the study of Krystal et al. (1994), there was nothing that could be classified as hallucinations. Nor, unlike what Krystal et al. (1994) and others had claimed, did any subjects show formal thought disorder (the only changes observed were vagueness and muddling of speech in two subjects which resembled the effects of intoxication). The single truly psychosis-like symptom was referential thinking, which 7 of the 15 subjects described. Some examples are shown in Box 6.1.

Box 6.1 Examples of Healthy Subjects' Descriptions of Referential Ideas on Ketamine (Pomarol-Clotet et al., 2006)

Volunteer 4

I feel so enclosed, I almost feel as though I'm in a cage or ... it's almost like a big brother type thing, people watching ... I know people aren't looking at me, but I feel as though people could be looking at me ... as though there's cameras or something like that.

Volunteer 5

Some of the questions when I was in the scanner, it was like they were saying one thing but what they're actually trying to do is discover what's going on somewhere else. People saying what they're supposed to say. People seem to be saying things for effect, instead of saying what they actually want. Some of the questions in the scanner seemed like they were specially put to make you think about something else. [As] if one's doing something for a reason but trying to make it look like they don't mean to do it. Things specially arranged beyond the experiment ... It's like someone wants you to think something and so they make you.

Volunteer 9

I feel they may talk about me. I think that they're thinking that I'm the centre of the world, although I know they're probably not. Laughing, not critical. I feel like a puppet, I feel guided by people around, to say things.

This volunteer also retrospectively described that she thought the interviewer was controlling her replies to questions by looking at her, and that people at the scanner were maybe spies; 'I was convinced'.

Volunteer 11

I feel paranoid that people are [looking at me] but I know that they're not, 'cause I'm in an experiment, so I know that they're not. I feel like I've not got control over what I'm saying, so I feel like what I am saying is not right, and then people are just looking at me and ... OK. I feel as if people's reactions are different to me, reacting differently to me, but I don't feel people are gossiping about me. They just seem to be giving me a lot more attention, a lot more time, everything seems a lot slower. It's like that film [The Truman Show].

I feel things have been specially arranged beyond the experiment. I've got that feeling but I know they haven't.

It feels like something's happening but I'm not quite sure what's going on. I don't quite know what it is.

I feel like I'm the focus, everyone is watching me, which obviously you are doing. I feel like there's more to it than what's actually happening. I feel like I'm not being told everything. Something going to happen and I haven't been told.

Volunteer 14

[During second (placebo) interview] I suppose I did [feel self-conscious during the first session]. Maybe people were looking at me longer than they would normally. A bit, definitely... I think it could have been because of my concentration – I couldn't really make out what they were saying, and so maybe I then thought they were talking about me, and maybe judging me, judging my reaction to it. At the time maybe I thought they were a bit critical.

Volunteer 15

It feels as if I'm on stage being watched by an audience. Things are not as they should be. People might be laughing at me because I'm not myself.

The unmistakable impression is of a phenomenon that appeared to be similar in all the subjects who experienced it, and went beyond what could be understood as simple ideas of reference. The account given by one of the subjects, who compared her experiences to a film, *The Truman Show* (whose plot revolves around a man who unknowingly is the main character in a soap-opera-like TV series) is particularly telling in this respect.

Ketamine may also be capable of also inducing propositional delusions, specifically the Capgras delusion. Corlett et al. (2010a) described a 26-year-old healthy volunteer who was given the drug intravenously who described that, 'every time you left the room, I thought another person dressed in your clothes was coming back into the room ... it wasn't scary, just another person dressed in your clothes, doing your job, but the person was a little older in age and weighed more'.

Glutamate: Not Just a Wiring Neurotransmitter

There is nothing mysterious about the function of glutamate – it is the brain's main excitatory neurotransmitter. Neurons that use it tend to be projection neurons (interneurons are mainly inhibitory, though excitatory ones using glutamate also exist), and they make up important pathways from the cortex to the basal ganglia, the thalamus, the brainstem and the spinal cord. Going in the opposite direction, the massive thalamo-cortical radiation is glutamatergic. Many cortico-cortical connections also use the transmitter. The pathway from the entorhinal cortex to the hippocampus, the perforant path, is glutamatergic, as are circuits within the hippocampus itself (Storm-Mathisen, 1981).

As a paradigmatic 'wiring' neurotransmitter, the role of glutamate is to enable the brain to perform the innumerable operations it happens to be engaged in at any given moment. As such, it seems difficult to see how a simple blockade of transmission, in line with the glutamate hypothesis of schizophrenia, could give rise to the kind of symptoms produced by phencyclidine and ketamine – the more likely result would be a progressive shutdown of cognitive and then all other brain functions. Fortunately for its role in delusions, however, this is not the whole story, because glutamate has another role, one which turns out to be mediated specifically by the NMDA receptor. In fact, it may well be that the NMDA receptor does not have very much to do at all with the actual task of transmitting an electrical signal from one neuron to the next.

It used to be believed that post-synaptic NMDA receptors and the other main class of fast or ionotropic post-synaptic glutamate receptor, the AMPA receptor (a third type of ionotropic receptor, the kianate receptor, has only a limited distribution in the brain), both participated equally in glutamatergic synaptic transmission. However, it has gradually become clear that this role is fulfilled principally by AMPA receptors (Citri & Malenka, 2008). In contrast, the main function of the NMDA receptor appears to be to induce long-term potentiation (LTP), a phenomenon that was first described in the hippocampus, but is now considered to be exhibited by virtually all synapses in the mammalian brain (Bliss & Collingridge, 1993; Malenka & Bear, 2004; Citri & Malenka, 2008). LTP takes the form of an abrupt increase in the intensity of post-synaptic activation which occurs in the wake of previous high frequency presynaptic stimulation. It typically lasts a few hours, although durations of days, weeks and up to a year have been documented (Abraham & Williams, 2003).

The main mechanism by which LTP is achieved involves so-called receptor trafficking, the production of new AMPA receptors which are then mobilized and inserted into the post-synaptic cell membrane (see Figure 6.2). In its later phases, the process also involves protein synthesis (Abrahamson & Williams, 2003) and in all probability the structural remodelling of dendritic spines (Bosch and Hayashi, 2012).

LTP is currently exciting great interest in neuroscience because it appears to be the predominant form of synaptic plasticity in the mammalian brain – changes in the strength or efficacy of transmission that take place as a result of previous activity at the synapse. As such, it may provide an answer to the puzzle of how the central nervous system performs one of its most important functions, that of storing information. Whether LTP, alone or in conjunction with other forms of synaptic plasticity, can be regarded as the biological basis of learning and memory does not yet have a definitive answer. However, evidence that it is necessary if not sufficient for these functions continues to accumulate (Martin et al., 2000; Takeuchi et al., 2014)

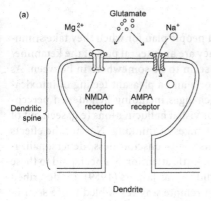

(a)

Molecules of glutamate bind to recognition sites on NMDA receptors as well as AMPA receptors. The ionotropic AMDA receptors admit sodium ions when activated, resulting in a moderate local depolarization...

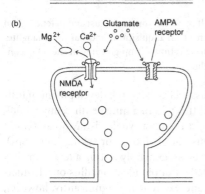

(b)

...that dislodges the magnesium ions blocking the NMDA receptors. Large quantities of calcium ions may now enter the neuron through the NMDA receptors' calcium channels. The calcium influx affects the metabolic machinery of the cell...

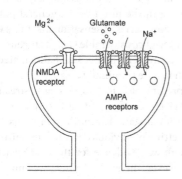

(c)

...resulting in the addition of more AMPA receptors to the postsynaptic membrane. The synapse has thus been strengthened and it will respond more rapidly and more strongly to future releases of glutamate.

Figure 6.2 AMPA receptor trafficking.
Source: Reproduced with permission from Breedlove, A. M. & Watson, N. V. (2013). *Biological Psychology: an Introduction to Behavioral, Cognitive and Clinical Neuroscience*, 7th Edition. Sunderland, MA: Sinauer Associates.

Cannabis

Unusual ideas and perceptual changes are not what people plan for when they take stimulant drugs like amphetamine. On the other hand they are an integral part of the ketamine/ phencyclidine experience. The effects of cannabis seem to lie somewhere in between. As described by Iversen (2008b), in addition to euphoria and a pleasant feeling of intoxication, people who take the drug describe sensory changes including heightened perception, perceptual distortions, synaesthesia and minor visual hallucinations (e.g. seen out of the corner of the eye), plus a range of subjective changes in thinking. Nor are the effects always pleasurable: some people experience intense self-consciousness, depersonalization, derealization and paranoia (Earleywine, 2002). Little attention has been paid to these latter effects in the literature, but one author who did so was Jaspers (1959). He described ideas of reference in hashish intoxication that in a remote way resembled those seen in schizophrenia.

> The intoxicated person feels defeated and finds himself in a situation of distrust and defence. Even the most banal question sounds like an examination or an inquisition, and harmless laughter sounds like derision. An accidental glance leads to the reaction – 'stop gawping at me'. One constantly sees menacing faces, one senses traps, hears allusions.

There is also a long tradition of cannabis being associated with the development of full-blown psychosis. One of the earliest descriptions of this was in a nineteenth century book on the potential medical uses of hashish written by a French psychiatrist, Moreau (1845) (also known as Moreau de Tours, apparently because of his liking for taking long trips). He described the occurrence of acute psychotic reactions, generally lasting a few hours but sometimes as long as a week, whose features included paranoid ideation, illusions, hallucinations, delusions, depersonalization, restlessness and excitement. Significantly, however, he also noted that there could be 'delirium, disorientation, and marked clouding of consciousness' (Moreau 1845, cited by D'Souza et al., 2004; Radhakrishnan et al, 2014).

By the second half of the twentieth century, the link between cannabis and serious mental disturbance had become firmly established, at least in the mind of the general public. Among other factors contributing to this perception were a series of sensationalist films with titles like *Reefer Madness* and *Devil's Harvest* which enjoyed considerable success throughout the 1930s, 1940s and 1950s. The former featured one character who became hallucinated on the drug and another who ended up in an institution for the criminally insane.

Meanwhile, in academic circles, a link was not proving easy to find. A steady stream of case reports and case series, reviewed by Thomas (1993), confirmed that taking cannabis, usually in high dosage, could cause an acute confusional state. Psychotic symptoms were prominent in these reports, but were present in the setting of obvious cognitive impairment and disorientation. Thomas (1993) also felt that there was evidence for the occurrence of schizophrenia-like states in clear consciousness. However, the evidence here was not altogether convincing since it depended on the one hand on case reports of psychosis where confusion was not mentioned (which does not mean that it was not present), and on the other on a handful of studies which documented the presence of cannabis in the urine of patients admitted to hospital with psychosis.

The association was finally established after a series of epidemiological surveys carried out between 1988 and 2002 (one of which was van Os et al.'s NEMESIS study described in Chapter 4) all found that regular cannabis use was a risk factor for the development of schizophrenia (see Arseneault et al., 2004). Even so, the increased risk turned out to be relatively small: according to a meta-analysis of these and other studies (Moore et al., 2007), the odds ratio for what the authors termed a psychotic outcome (which included both clinically diagnosed psychosis and the presence of psychotic or psychotic-like experiences) was 1.4, rising to 2.09 among the heaviest users.

The time was now right for an experimental study of the acute psychosis-inducing effects of cannabis on volunteers of the kind carried out with ketamine. D'Souza et al. (2004) gave 22 non-dependent cannabis users with no history of psychiatric disorder intravenous tetrahydrocannabinol, the main psychoactive component of cannabis, or placebo (ethanol) under double-blind conditions. While on the drug, the subjects rated themselves as experiencing anxiety, changed perception of time, feelings of unreality and various alterations in perception and thinking. The effects peaked at around ten minutes and returned to baseline levels after around three hours. Importantly, the authors gave examples of the subjects' descriptions of their experiences, and these are shown in Box 6.2. It can be seen that these included referentiality and suspiciousness, with statements that seem closely similar to those made by the subjects in Pomarol-Clotet et al.'s (2006) study of ketamine. Heightened perception was also described. Statements that D'Souza et al. (2004) placed under the heading of 'conceptual disorganization, thought disorder, thought blocking, loosening of associations', were actually descriptions of subjective changes in thinking rather than objectively rated formal thought disorder.

Box 6.2 Experiences Described by Healthy Volunteers Given Intravenous Tetrahydrocannabinol (Reproduced with permission from D'Souza et al., 2004)

Suspiciousness/Paranoia

I thought you could read my mind, that's why I didn't answer.
I thought you all were trying to trick me by changing the rules of the tests to make me fail.
I thought you were turning the clock back to confuse me.
I could hear someone on typing on the computer... and I thought you all were trying to program me.
I felt as if my mind was nude.
I thought you all were giving me THC thru the BP machine and the sheets.

Loss of Insight

I thought that this was real ... I was convinced this wasn't an experiment.

Conceptual Disorganization, Thought Disorder, Thought Blocking, Loosening of Associations

I couldn't keep track of my thoughts ... they'd suddenly disappear.
It seemed as if all the questions were coming to me at once ... everything was happening in staccato.
My thoughts were fragmented ... the past present and future all seemed to be happening at once.

Grandiosity

I felt I could see into the future ... I thought I was God.

Inability to Filter Out Irrelevant Background Stimuli

The air conditioning that I couldn't hear before suddenly became deafening. I thought I could hear the dripping of the i.v. and it was louder than your voice.

The Brain's Endocannabinoid System

How cannabis exerted its psychological effects was a complete mystery until the late 1980s when neuronal receptors for a synthetic tetrahydrocannabinol-like compound were discovered (see Wilson & Nicoll, 2002; Kano et al., 2009). These cannabinoid receptors, known as CB1 receptors to distinguish them from CB2 receptors which are located on immune system cells, are now known to be abundant in the brain and are present at particularly high levels in the frontal and anterior cingulate cortex, the basal ganglia, the hippocampus, the hypothalamus and the cerebellum. They are mainly localized to axons and nerve terminals, and tetrohydrocannabinol has stimulatory effects at them. The first endogenous ligand to be identified for CB1 receptors was N-arachidonylethanolamide, and was given the name anandamide after the Sanskrit word for bliss. A second ligand, 2-arachidonylglycerol (known rather more prosaically as 2-AG) has since been identified and is probably the main natural transmitter.

The brain's endocannabinoid system is different again from the dopamine and glutamate systems. In fact it is not really a system at all in the sense of being a neuronal pathway with cell bodies, axons and synaptic terminals. As described by Iversen (2003), anandamide and 2-AG are synthesized by postsynaptic neurons in response to strong presynaptic activity. The transmitters are then released into the extracellular space where they diffuse back across the synapse and interact with CB1 receptors localized on axon terminals. Because the signal is spread simply by diffusion it influences hundreds of synaptic terminals in a region approximately 40 micrometres (0.04 mm) in diameter. Its effect is to reduce activity for a period of time lasting tens of seconds in both excitatory and inhibitory neurons. In other words the endocannabinoid system is a rapid, locally acting retrograde signalling mechanism with volume characteristics.

In 2001 it was shown that that endocannabinoid signalling is the physiological basis for a phenomenon that had been discovered some years previously, depolarization-induced suppression of inhibition (Wilson & Nicoll, 2001). This is a transient reduction of inhibitory synaptic transmission that occurs when postsynaptic neurons are depolarized. As it acts on inhibitory neurons, its net effect is excitatory. A complementary effect on excitatory neurons, depolarization-induced suppression of excitation, also appears to depend on endocannabinoid transmission (Kreitzer & Regehr, 2001). Since they change neuronal activity on the basis of previous experience, depolarization-induced suppression of inhibition and excitation are forms of synaptic plasticity. There is evidence that endocannabinoids are involved in longer-term forms of synaptic plasticity as well (Kano et al., 2009; Kano, 2014). These appear to include particularly long-term depression (LTD), the reverse of LTP, where high intensity stimulation of a presynaptic neuron results in long-lasting reduced efficacy of synaptic transmission (Citri and Malenka, 2008).

Conclusion: Fitting the Neurochemical Pieces Together

The facts are clear: when brain chemistry is interfered with in certain specific ways, delusions are the result. Beyond this, however, confusion mostly seems to reign. Dopamine, glutamate and endocannabinoids are neurotransmitters with very different modes of action which perform very different functions in the brain. Stimulant drugs cause delusions as part of their ability to induce a general schizophrenia-like state; on the other hand the only truly psychosis-like symptom that ketamine and cannabis seem to be associated with, at least under experimental conditions, is referential (and possibly also propositional) delusions. Probably only around half of individuals who abuse stimulants will ever experience any kind of psychotic symptoms, but referential delusions seem to occur with substantial frequency after a single intravenous dose of ketamine or cannabis. The evidence is clearly not telling a simple story, but maybe it is not an impenetrable maze either.

The most popular way to try to bring order to the findings has been to assert the primacy of one transmitter. This transmitter is often dopamine, no doubt reflecting the central role it has played and continues to play in schizophrenia research. Supporters of this position face difficulties in trying to explain why delusions are not an immediate effect of stimulant drugs, and why not everyone develops them even after repeated exposure, but these are not insurmountable obstacles. A bigger stumbling block is that, in order to explain how NMDA receptor antagonist drugs can also produce delusions, some kind of reciprocal interaction between dopamine and glutamate usually ends up being invoked. Yet, as this chapter has shown, this is not in any sense an accurate description of the respective roles of these two neurotransmitters.

It does not take long to realize that casting glutamate as the villain of the piece will run into the same kind of problems, and probably others as well. A better approach might therefore be to focus on what dopamine and glutamate have in common. At first sight the gulf between the two seems to be huge: dopamine is a volume transmitter with well-established behavioural functions, whereas glutamate is the epitome of a wiring neurotransmitter. Glutamate, however, turns out to have a second role, that of mediating LTP, and this is in a certain sense modulatory (although it does not depend on volume transmission). In fact, it seems that the NMDA receptor makes little or no direct contribution to the actual transmission that takes place across glutamatergic synapses, a point that seems to have mostly escaped schizophrenia researchers to date.

Being able to argue that what gives neurotransmitters delusion-inducing properties is the fact that they are modulatory is not by itself very enlightening. However, when what is known about the endocannabinoid system is added to the equation, something more concrete starts to take shape. This is that all three transmitters appear to play roles in what might be referred to as how the brain records experience. In the case of dopamine, the link is explicitly with learning. For the other two transmitters it is their involvement in synaptic plasticity, which may or may not be the ultimate basis of memory. In this way, the neurochemical evidence might finally lead to a hypothesis, that delusions represent a derangement in the neurochemical processes underlying learning and memory. The idea that memory might be relevant to delusions surfaces again in a minor way in the next chapter. The concept of delusions being due to a derangement in the mechanisms of reinforcement-based learning has more direct implications – it is essentially the salience theory of delusions, which is discussed in detail in Chapter 8.

Delusion-like Phenomena in Neurological Disease

Delusions, as well as certain other symptoms that bear a more than passing resemblance to them, are sometimes seen in patients with neurological disorders. As noted in Chapter 5, the fact that this occurs has the potential to inject some much-needed fresh thinking into the psychology of delusions. However, as noted in the same chapter, these states tend to develop in the context of strokes and other disorders that cause brain damage and so challenge the view that delusions are unrelated to psychological deficits. Whether they really do violate this principle or whether they are simply the exception that proves the rule is therefore something that needs to be considered carefully.

Before going any further, however, two red herrings need to be identified and dealt with. The first is that some of the delusions seen in neurological patients form part of a wider psychiatric disturbance. Thus, schizophrenia is well-established as being over-represented in epilepsy, traumatic brain injury and several other central nervous system diseases (Davison & Bagley, 1969; David & Prince, 2005; Clancy et al., 2014). There is also an increased frequency of delusional disorder in multiple sclerosis (Ron & Logsdail, 1989). Strokes and Parkinson's disease are clinically associated with depression and in some cases it seems likely that this will show psychotic features. There does not seem to be any way that these so-called secondary or symptomatic presentations can be informative about underlying mechanisms of delusions specifically, since the abnormal beliefs are usually just one symptom among many. To be of interest from this point of view, the delusion or delusion-like phenomenon needs to occur in isolation – or be 'monothematic' in the terminology used by those working in this field.

Two other disorders, delirium and dementia, present another set of problems. Delirium, or the acute confusional state, is a regular response to almost all forms of acute brain injury and to systemic illnesses that can affect brain function. Along with cognitive impairment, which characteristically fluctuates, many patients show delusions, dream-like hallucinatory experiences and rambling incoherent speech. Although the delusions of delirium are often instantly recognizable as such, being crude, fleeting and fragmentary, this is not always the case and sometimes they can quite well formed and complex (Cutting, 1980). Patients with dementia not infrequently develop ideas about being robbed, or that their reflection in a mirror is another person, or that people have moved into their house. As Lishman (1998) pointed out, such beliefs are delusions only in the technical sense, in that they are held because the evidence to the contrary is not understood, not because it is rejected. However, it is also recognized that beliefs that go further into the realm of true delusions can also occur, especially in the early stages of the disorder. In any event, if the aim is to show that delusions can be the result of a disturbance in one or more specific cognitive systems, it is probably not a good idea to rely on evidence from these two disorders, which by definition affect brain function generally.

So, after making sure that the relevant phenomena are monothematic and excluding anything that raises the suspicion of being the product of delirium or dementia, there are three types of neurological symptom that can be considered delusion-like. In approximate reverse order of similarity to delusions, these are anosognosia for hemiplegia, where the patient believes he or she can move a limb that is paralysed; confabulation, which everyone agrees is different from delusions, but turns out to share a surprising number of features with them; and finally the Capgras syndrome, something that is unquestionably a delusion, but which in all probability occurs in neurological patients at least as frequently as it does in patients with schizophrenia.

Anosognosia for Hemiplegia

This first delusion-like phenomenon was originally described by the French neurologist Babinski (1914, 1918). He gave a description of two patients who had had strokes but showed an unawareness of their paralysis amounting to complete denial. Critchley (1953) summarized his account as follows:

> The first patient was a woman had been paralyzed down the left side for years, but who never mentioned the fact. If asked to move the affected limb she remained immobile and silent, behaving as though the question had been put to someone else. Babinski's second patient was a victim of left hemiplegia. Whenever she was asked about what was the matter with her, she talked about her backache, or her phlebitis, but never once did she refer to her powerless left arm. When told to move that limb, she did nothing and said nothing, or else a mere 'Voilà, c'est fait!' During a consultation, when her doctors were discussing the merits of physiotherapy in her presence, she broke in … 'Why should I have electrical treatment? I am not paralyzed.'

The paralysis was left-sided in both cases and Babinski (1914, 1918) wondered if anosognosia might therefore be specific to lesions of the right hemisphere. He also drew attention to the fact that the both the patients had sensory impairment in the affected limbs, presciently as it turned out.

Further case reports followed and there is now a substantial body of literature on the disorder. It usually occurs with strokes, although it is also seen following head injury and after surgery for tumours (Weinstein & Kahn, 1955; Cocchini et al., 2002). As Babinski suspected, it is almost always seen in patients with left-sided paralysis. The denial of paralysis is typically noted in the immediate aftermath of the stroke or brain injury and often improves over a matter of days. However, as was the case in Babinski's first patient, it can sometimes become chronic, although this is uncommon.

At first sight, anosognosia for hemiplegia does not seem to be especially relevant to delusions; if anything it seems more closely related to the lack of insight seen in schizophrenia. What makes the link with delusions more compelling, however, is the fact that in many cases the patients are not just unaware of their paralysis but actively deny it and in the process make quite brazen false statements. The neuropsychologist Ramachandran's (1996) description of such a case, written in his typical lively style, is reproduced in Box 7.1.

Box 7.1 A Case of Anosognosia (Reproduced with permission from Ramachandran, 1996)

Mrs. F.D. was a patient in her late 70s who had sustained a stroke about I week prior to my seeing her in the hospital. The left side other body was completely paralyzed as a result of her stroke. I walked into the hospital and started chatting with her.

V.S.R.: Mrs. F.D., why did you come to the hospital?
F.D.: I came here because I had a stroke.
V.S.R.: When did you have the stroke?
F.D.: A week ago.
V.S.R: How do you know you had a stroke?
F.D.: I know I had a stroke because I fell in the bathroom and my daughter then brought me to the hospital and they did some brain scans and told me I had a stroke.

Clearly, she was aware she had a stroke.

V.S.R.: Mrs. F.D., how are you feeling today?
F.D.: I've got a headache. I've had a stroke so they brought me to the hospital.
V.S.R.: Mrs. F.D., can you walk?
F.D.: Yes.

She had been in a wheelchair for the past week. She could not walk.

V.S.R.: Mrs. F.D. hold out your hands. Can you move your hands?
F.D.: Yes.
V.S.R.: Can you use your right hand?
F.D.: Yes.
V.S.R.: Can you use your left hand?
F.D.: Yes.
V.S.R.: Are both hands equally strong?
F.D.: Yes, of course they are.
V.S.R.: Can you point to my nose with your right hand?

She pointed to my nose.

V.S.R.: Point to me with your left hand.

Her hand lay paralyzed in front of her.

V.S.R.: Are you pointing at my nose?
F.D.: Yes.
V.S.R.: Can you clearly see it pointing?
F.D.: Yes, it is about 2 inches from your nose.

At this point the woman produced a frank confabulation, a delusion about the position of her arm. She had no problems with her vision and could see her arm perfectly clearly, yet she created a delusion about her own body image. I couldn't resist asking her:

V.S.R.: Can you clap?
F.D.: Of course I can clap.
V.S.R.: Will you clap for me?

She proceeded to make clapping movements with her right hand as if clapping with an imaginary hand near the midline.

V.S.R.: Are you clapping?
F.D.: Yes, I'm clapping.

Thus, here at last, we may have an answer to the Zen master's eternal riddle: What is the sound of one hand clapping? Mrs. F.D. obviously knew the answer!

While one might quibble with Ramachandran's use of the word delusion in this patient, in others the term becomes harder to avoid. A patient described by Sandifer (1946), when asked if her paralysed hand was hers, replied 'Not mine, doctor.' When then asked whose hand it was, she stated, 'I suppose it's yours, doctor,' and went on to suggest that the ring on it was the doctor's as well. Other patients have suggested that their arm belonged to a previous occupant of the hospital bed or that it might have been left in the ambulance that brought them to hospital (Bisiach & Geminiani, 1991). In what may or may not be a phenomenon related to anosognosia, patients even occasionally develop the belief that they have a third arm or leg. Halligan and co-workers (Halligan et al., 1993; Halligan & Marshall, 1995) described two such patients with left-sided strokes in whom such a belief persisted for several months. Both were lucid and realized that others would find what they said unbelievable. The first patient had well-preserved general intellectual function, but he became noticeably muddled when he went into detail about the extra limb, saying at times that it was artificial or that it had been amputated.

Strange as it now seems, for a long time the dominant explanatory paradigm for anosognosia was psychodynamic. The originator of this theory was an American neurologist, Weinstein, who, together with a colleague (Weinstein and Kahn, 1950, 1955), carried out a study in which they investigated the life histories of patients who developed anosognosia. They claimed to have found evidence that the symptom developed in individuals who were constitutionally prone to use the Freudian defence mechanism of denial. Later, Weinstein (1970) held up as an example the case of Woodrow Wilson, who felt himself perfectly capable of carrying on as president of the United States and considered seeking re-election for a third term, despite having suffered a stroke which left him very severely disabled.

After the collapse of psychoanalysis in America in the late 1970s (see Chapter 3), more reality based theories began to appear. One of these grew out of the observation that anosognosia seemed to occur exclusively in patients with left-sided strokes. Perhaps, therefore, it was a consequence of disturbed functioning of the right hemisphere. However, there was a problem with this proposal: patients with right-sided strokes often have aphasia, which would effectively prevent them from describing anosognosia if they had it. Cutting (1978), a psychiatrist with a lifelong interest in the brain bases of psychotic symptoms, examined this possibility in a survey of 100 patients with recent strokes. He found that 28 of the 48 with a left-sided stroke denied the presence of weakness when asked about it. Thirty of the 52 who had had a right-sided stroke were so aphasic that they could not answer questions about anosognosic symptoms. Among the remaining 22, 3 denied the existence of their paralysis and a further 9 showed phenomena commonly associated with anosognosia such as minimizing the importance of the weakness or stating that the limb did not belong to them.

The starting point for the other main class of theories of anosognosia was also one of Babinski's (1914, 1918) original observations, that patients with anosognosia also show sensory impairment in the affected limb. This finding has been amply confirmed by later studies, for example being found to be present in 87 per cent of the patients with anosognosia in Cutting's (1978) series. In its simple form, the argument goes as follows: if a patient just has paralysis, trying to move the limb will result in somatosensory feedback communicating the fact that the limb has not moved. If, however, there is also sensory loss in the limb, the patient will not register the fact that the limb has failed to move and so will fail to realize that he or she is actually paralysed. There are several variations on this theme, which invoke central mechanisms like corollary discharge and predictive modelling (Bisiach & Geminiani, 1991; Frith et al., 2000), but the principle is always the same – at some level there is a failure to detect that an intended movement has not taken place, and this prevents the patient from realizing that the limb is paralysed.

While theories of this second type provide a plausible basis for what might be termed the basic anosognosic experience, they still face the problem of why the belief persists despite what is, quite literally, the evidence of the patients' own eyes. As Ramachandran (1996) put it, 'it is the vehemence of the denial, not merely the indifference to the paralysis, that cries out for an explanation'. Clearly, something more (and hopefully not psychodynamic) is needed to make the theory work. Davies et al. (2005), examined the different possibilities for what this additional factor might be, in an article whose authors included Coltheart, someone who will figure prominently in rest of this chapter.

The first candidate Davies et al. (2005) considered was cognitive impairment. Anosognosia is, as noted previously, typically an acute phenomenon, occurring in the days following a stroke when confusion and disorientation are common, and in many cases the patient will have recently emerged from a period of unconsciousness. For example, Sandifer's (1946) patient showed denial of paralysis just two days after suffering a stroke and she died shortly afterwards. Ramachandran's (1996) patient FD had had a stroke only a week previously, and while he established that she was oriented, this did not mean that lesser and/or fluctuating degrees of confusion were necessarily absent. At first sight, the evidence in favour of this proposal seems strong: three clinical series of anosognosic patients (Nathanson et al., 1952; Ullman, 1962; Weinstein & Kahn, 1955) reported that disorientation was present in all cases, and a fourth (Gross & Kaltenback, 1955) found that 18 per cent were oriented but still showed a 'lack of critical awareness of surroundings'. However, going against these findings, Cutting (1978) found that while 22 of the patients in his survey who showed anosognosia and could be questioned were disoriented, 9 were not. Four of these latter patients showed evidence of memory impairment, but this still left 5 who developed the syndrome in apparently clear consciousness. Davies et al. (2005) also cited a number of studies which found no association between the level of cognitive impairment and presence or absence of anosognosia. But the strongest piece of evidence against the cognitive impairment theory is that anosognosia sometimes outlasts any credible period of post-stroke confusion. The stroke in one of Babinski's two original cases had happened four years previously, and at least two other well-documented cases of chronic anosognosia have since been published (House & Hodges, 1988; Cocchini et al., 2002).

Davies et al. (2005) then considered a second possibility, which seemed on the face of it highly plausible. This was neglect, a syndrome where patients who have had strokes show lack of attention to the affected side of their body and/or the environment on that side, for example only shaving or putting on makeup on one side, or only drawing one half of a picture of a man or a clock. Nevertheless, although patients with anosognosia commonly also show neglect, Davies et al. (2005) were able to find several studies which demonstrated a double dissociation between the two – there are patients who show neglect without anosognosia and others who show anosognosia without neglect.

With the obvious suspects eliminated, Davies et al. (2005) were forced to conclude that the additional factor was some other, as yet undefined cognitive abnormality. They had little to say about what this abnormality might be, but they speculated that it might involve updating of knowledge and beliefs in the light of information from different sources. They also added the rider that, while it seemed to represent an impairment, it was one that could apparently sometimes occur 'without any apparent departure from cognitive normality'.

Confabulation

Although the term confabulation is often employed in a loose way – for example Ramachandran (1996) used it to describe his anosognosic patient's attempts to rationalize her inability to move her arm – it strictly refers to the tendency of patients with amnesia to produce false memories. Sometimes this occurs only when the patient is asked questions, but in other cases it is spontaneous, taking the form of 'a persistent unprovoked outpouring of erroneous memories' (Kopelman, 2010). The neurological disorder in which confabulation classically occurs is the Wernicke-Korsakoff syndrome, a consequence of brain damage due to thiamine deficiency which is seen particularly in alcoholics. Another common cause is rupture of an aneurysm in the anterior communicating artery, which supplies large parts of the frontal lobes. It can also be seen in the early stages of dementia, a presentation that is (or used to be) referred to as 'presbyophrenia'. Finally, it is an occasional complication of other disorders such as multiple sclerosis and herpes simplex encephalitis.

Being a pathology of memory, confabulation does not seem on the face of it to have any obvious connection with delusions, except perhaps in the special case of delusional memories. However, closer inspection reveals that it shows several features that make it 'interestingly belief-like' to borrow a phrase from Bayne and Pacherie (2005). One of these is that the events confabulating patients relate are often highly unlikely and at times impossible. For example, Turner and Coltheart (2010) described how their patient GN once told them that he had gone to a party the night before where he met a woman with a bee's head. On other occasions he stated that he was in hospital because he had been attacked by enemy aircraft when boarding a submarine, that he had been bitten by a rabbit, and that a gunfight had just taken place involving communists who were trying take over the nearby National Archive Centre. Another patient (Damasio et al., 1985) stated he was a space pirate at the time of the Columbia space mission. The patient reported by Metcalf et al. (2007) described how his father, who had not visited the previous weekend, had failed to do so because he had been abducted by aliens.

Confabulations are typically fleeting and change each time the patient produces them. This, however, may also not be as great a point of difference from delusions as might be thought. Just as delusions – especially delusional memories – are not always fixed and unchanging, there is a long if somewhat intangible tradition of confabulations sometimes becoming entrenched. Korsakoff himself (quoted by Berrios, 1998) commented that, '[o]n occasions, such patients invent some fiction and constantly repeat it, so that a peculiar delirium develops, rooted in false recollections' (according to Berrios, by delirium Korsakoff almost certainly meant delusion). In the contemporary literature Turner and Coltheart (2010) drew attention to the confabulating patient described by Burgess and McNeil (1999) who started every day expressing the belief that he had to conduct a stock take at a local shop. Similarly, a patient of Mattioli et al. (1999) would consistently awake with the belief that he was a schoolboy and had to attend a swimming carnival at school – despite being 36 years old and unable to walk. Kopelman (2010) reported a patient who was described as being stuck in the 1970s or early 1980s, thinking Margaret Thatcher was prime minister and Richard Nixon was the president of the United States (this was despite the fact that their terms of office did not actually overlap).

Do confabulations show the further delusion-like quality of being held with fixed, unshakeable conviction? This question is more controversial: Turner and Coltheart (2010) acknowledged that patients often seem happy to abandon their confabulations and replace them with others. On the other hand, they and other authors (Moscovitch, 1995; Gilboa & Verfaellie, 2010; Langdon & Bayne, 2010) have been impressed by the apparent sincerity with which confabulations are expressed and the fact that patients not infrequently act on them, for example attempting to leave the hospital on some errand they believe they have to do, or doing things that reflect a belief that the hospital is actually their place of work. What seems undeniable is that when confabulating patients are confronted with the all too obvious contradictions in what they say, they often come up with what Turner and Coltheart (2010) called secondary claims, glib and frequently illogical rationalizations which put one in mind of anosognosia, and also with the kind of evidence that deluded patients sometimes produce with when asked to justify their beliefs. Thus, Mattioli et al.'s (1999) patient referred to above, when challenged about a statement that he had gone swimming in a lake the day before even though it was actually winter and he was significantly physically disabled, replied by saying 'But this is an especially mild January' and 'I still work, although I am sometimes a little tired.' Another, more elaborate example is shown in Box 7.2.

Box 7.2 How Confabulating Patients Justify Their Claims (Reproduced with permission from Moscovitch, 1995)

Patient HW was a 61-year-old man who had had a subarachnoid haemorrhage. Clipping near the anterior communicating artery resulted in widespread frontal ischaemia and infarction. The following is part of an interview that took place three years later.

Q. How long have you been married?
A. About 4 months.
Q. What's your wife's name?
A. Martha.
Q. How many children do you have?
A. Four. (He laughs.) Not bad for 4 months!
Q. How old are your children?
A. The eldest is 32, his name is Bob, and the youngest is 22, his name is Joe. (These answers are close to the actual age of the boys).
Q. (He laughs again.) How did you get these children in 4 months?
A. They're adopted.
Q. Who adopted them?
A. Martha and I.
Q. Immediately after you got married you wanted to adopt these older children?
A. Before we were married we adopted one of them, two of them. The eldest girl Brenda and Bob, and Joe and Dina since we were married.
Q. Does it all sound a little strange to you, what you are saying?
A. (He laughs.) I think it is a little strange.

In terms of the underlying cognitive mechanisms of confabulation, it is well established that memory impairment alone is not sufficient to produce it. Most amnesic patients do not confabulate and in those that do the symptom tends to disappear over time even if there is no improvement in memory. Clearly, something else needs to be present and according to an impressive list of studies this is impaired executive function (Mercer et al., 1977; Stuss et al.,

1978; Kapur & Coughlan, 1980; Baddeley & Wilson, 1988; DeLuca, 1993; Fischer et al., 1995; Hashimoto et al., 2000). This neuropsychological evidence is complemented by neuroanatomical findings which have linked confabulation to lesions in the frontal lobe, particularly a discrete subregion of this in the medial and orbitofrontal cortex, and perhaps also the left lateral prefrontal cortex (Gilboa & Moscovitch, 2002; Turner et al., 2008).

Despite some outstanding questions – not least the fact that patients with both memory and executive impairment do not necessarily show confabulation – these findings have given birth to a powerful cognitive neuropsychological theory of the symptom. This is the strategic retrieval account of Moscovitch and co-workers (Moscovitch, 1992, 1995; Moscovitch & Melo, 1997; Gilboa & Moscovitch 2002; Gilboa et al., 2006) which, along with another closely similar proposal (Burgess & Shallice, 1996), is currently the most influential approach to confabulation. Its central idea is that recall of a memory is an active, reconstructive act that depends on several different processes. The first of these is an associative mechanism whereby a retrieval cue interacts automatically with a stored memory trace in order to activate a representation of the original experience. Such a process is a feature of many if not all physiological theories of memory and is presumed to involve the hippocampus and other structures implicated in the amnesic syndrome. It is also a key part of Tulving's (1983) influential cognitive theory of memory, where it is referred to as synergistic ecphory, to highlight the fact that a combination between the cue and the stored representation takes place.

Once a memory trace has been activated by a cue, more strategic monitoring processes of the type associated with the prefrontal cortex are brought into play. As Moscovitch et al. (1992) put it:

> [T]he frontal lobes are necessary for converting remembering from a stupid reflexive act triggered by a cue to a reflective goal-directed activity that is under voluntary control. In trying to place a person that looks familiar to you or to determine where you were during the last week of July, the appropriate memory does not emerge automatically but must be ferreted out, often laboriously, by retrieval strategies.

One process that occurs at this stage is a kind of rapid and intuitive checking that assigns a 'feeling of rightness' to the retrieved memory. The site where this takes place is often identified as the ventromedial prefrontal cortex. There is much left unsaid about what exactly underlies feeling of rightness, but it is presumed to involve elements of familiarity and the emotional feelings the memory evokes. It is also considered to equate to the intrinsic sense of veridicality that often accompanies the successful recall of an event – I am often completely sure about what I had for breakfast this morning or where I went on holiday last year, even though I have no other basis for being so other than the fact that I remember the events concerned.

After a memory passes the feeling of rightness test it is then subjected to a slower, more deliberate checking process (or possibly the two processes take place at the same time). This second process is proposed to depend on the dorsolateral prefrontal cortex and it aims to decide by means of conflict detection and problem solving whether what has been retrieved is compatible with what was trying to be remembered, and also with other relevant memories and knowledge. It can override feeling of rightness but cannot change it. Importantly, this process is also engaged when the initial cue dependent ecphoric process fails, as it often does. In this case, a deliberate search process is initiated whose aim among other things is to

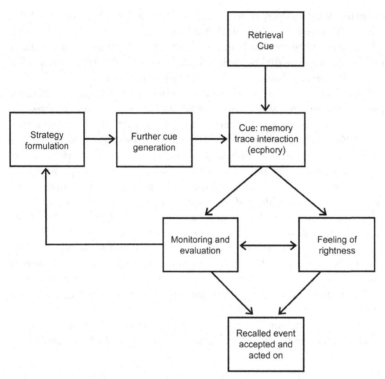

Figure 7.1 The strategic retrieval model of memory.
Source: Adapted from Gilboa, A., Alain, C., Stuss, D. T., Melo, B., Miller, S., & Moscovitch, M. (2006). Mechanisms of spontaneous confabulations: a strategic retrieval account. *Brain*, 129, 1399–1414. Reproduced with permission.

generate further potential retrieval cues. A diagram of the whole strategic retrieval model is shown in Figure 7.1.

According to the strategic retrieval theory, confabulation occurs when there is (a) a failure of memory cues to ecphorize memories due to disease affecting the hippocampus or other parts of the associative memory system; and (b) a failure of one or both of strategic monitoring processes, caused by incidental damage to other brain regions, especially the frontal lobes. This results in the patient failing to reject incorrect memories that are activated. (Such activation of incorrect memories may occur because the retrieval cue has been nonspecific enough to activate several potential memory traces, or alternatively because when synergistic ecphory does not work properly it produces errors of commission as well as of omission.) The problem is compounded by the patient failing to mount an orderly search for further cues when the initial direct associative cue fails to produce a result, which leads to further incorrect memories being activated and not rejected.

As with anosnognosia for hemiplegia, the strategic retrieval account of confabulation is a two factor theory. On the one hand there is a tendency to ecphorize erroneous memories, and on the other there is failure in a mechanism (or in this case two mechanisms) that prevents these memories being uncritically accepted. This point was not lost on Coltheart and co-workers (Metcalf et al., 2007; Turner & Coltheart, 2010) who speculated that the checking processes that make up the second factor might not be restricted just to the domain of memory, but might be a requirement for all information that enters conscious awareness.

The Capgras Syndrome

While confabulation and anosognosia for hemiplegia are at best only crude neurological approximations to delusions, there is no question that the Capgras syndrome is a fully fledged delusional belief. This can be stated with some confidence because for a long time it was believed to a purely psychiatric symptom, albeit a rare and exotic one.

Capgras' original description of the syndrome (see Ellis et al., 1994) was in a patient with a very florid psychosis, who among other things believed that her husband, daughters, neighbours and other acquaintances were being replaced by multiple doubles on an ongoing basis. His second patient and all the subsequent cases that were brought together by Enoch and co-workers (1967) in the first edition of their book *Uncommon Psychiatric Syndromes* had diagnoses of schizophrenia or paranoid psychosis, or in a few cases major affective disorder. What Enoch et al. (1967) wrote about the cause of the disorder drew heavily on psychoanalytic concepts, and contained no hint of what, neurologically speaking, was to come.

The tide began to turn only a year later when Gluckman (1968) reported a Capgras patient who showed evidence of cerebral atrophy, although the author still considered the diagnosis to be fundamentally one of schizophrenia. Three years later Weston and Whitlock (1971) described a 20-year-old man who sustained a serious head injury in a car accident and was left with multiple neuropsychological deficits. Within a few months he began to refer to his mother as 'that old woman who looks after me', explaining that his family had been killed by Chinese communists and that the people now claiming to be his parents and siblings were impostors. His condition improved slowly but five months later he remained doubtful whether his parents really were who they appeared to be.

Many more neurological cases of the Capgras syndrome have since been reported. In a review of these, Edelstyn and Obeyode (1999) found that it could occur in association with dementia, head trauma, epilepsy, cerebrovascular disease, brain tumours, multiple sclerosis and viral encephalitis, as well as a range of systemic diseases affecting brain function. Two clinical variants of the Capgras syndrome, the Fregoli syndrome, where the patient believes that the same person is disguising him/herself as different people, and intermetamorphosis, where people around the patient are believed to be constantly transforming into others, have also been reported in association with neurological disease (de Pauw et al., 1987; Burgess et al., 1996; Box et al., 1999; Feinberg et al., 1999).

Perusal of the individual case reports reveals that several of the patients also had other delusions and/or hallucinations and so are probably best regarded as cases of symptomatic schizophrenia. In others there was obvious evidence of confusion. Although some of the cases occurring in the context of dementia were convincing, in others there was room to wonder whether what was being described was simply a rationalization of the progressive failure to recognize friends and family that occurs with this condition. The minority of cases where the delusion was not part of a diagnosable psychotic syndrome, and where the patient was not obviously delirious or demented are summarized in Table 7.1. One or two of them are still open to question, for example, the patient reported by Alexander et al. (1979): he developed what was apparently an isolated Capgras delusion after a serious head injury, but he had been clearly psychotic in the months leading up to his accident (which was caused by his erratic behaviour). In several more cases, the absence of other psychiatric symptoms was

Table 7.1 Neurological Cases of Capgras Syndrome Excluding Patients with Symptomatic Schizophrenia, Delirium and Dementia

Study	Patient's Details	Brain Pathology	Other Symptoms	Other Symptoms	Duration	Comments
Weston and Whitlock (1971)	Male, 20	Head injury	-		7 months	-
MacCallum case 2 (1973)	Female, 28	?Stroke ?Basilar migraine	Believed that she was going to be poisoned. Abnormal attitude to paralysed right side.		3 weeks	-
Staton et al. (1982)	Male, 31	Head injury	Reduplication of place, time and self.		4 years	-
Bhatia (1990)	Female, 35	Migraine	-	Other schizophrenic symptoms stated to be absent	3 weeks	Migraine symptoms recovered after 2 days but the Capgras delusion lasted longer.
Förstl et al. (1994)	Female, 33	Subarachnoid haemorrhage	Not sure if she was herself or somebody else. Sometimes felt she was the object of an evil experiment.		Unstated (months)	-
Lebert et al. (1994)	Female, 40	Multiple sclerosis	-		Multiple episodes lasting 3–4 weeks	Most delusional episodes coincided with attacks of demyelination.
Hirstein and Ramachandran (1997)	Male, 30	Head injury	Reduplication of place and self.		2 years	-
Mattioli et al. (1999)	Male, 51	Head injury	Confabulation. Reduplication of place and possibly time. Anosognosia immediately after head injury.		At least 2 years	Did not explicitly claim that his wife was an impostor, only that she was someone else.

not spelt out as fully as might be wished. But overall, the occurrence of the Capgras delusion in monothematic form in several different neurological disease states can be regarded as reasonably well established.

It is also interesting to note that two of the patients in Table 7.1 additionally showed confabulation, and one had experienced anosognosia immediately after his head injury. Another patient, who developed a Capgras delusion in association with migraine, was described as having an abnormal attitude to the temporary paralysis of her right side that also occurred during the attack.

Any lingering doubts that the Capgras syndrome can arise monothematically in the context of neurological disease are laid to rest when it is realized that it is only one of a series of other reduplication or misidentification syndromes recognized in neurology. One such syndrome is reduplicative paramnesia, where patients believe that they are in another place which closely resembles the one they are actually in. For example, a head-injury patient described by Benson et al. (1976), although otherwise fully oriented, felt he was not in the Jamaica Plain Veterans Hospital in Boston but instead in another hospital with the same name in Taunton, Massachusetts, his home town. He acknowledged that Jamaica Plain was part of Boston and admitted it would be strange for there to be two Jamaica Plain Veterans Hospitals. Nevertheless, he insisted that this was the case. Another patient (Kapur et al., 1988), who was ultimately found to have suffered a minor right-sided stroke, went missing after visiting a friend. When he eventually arrived home he insisted that the house was not his, and he remarked on what a striking coincidence it was that the owners of this house had the same ornaments as he had in his house and kept similar items beside the bed.

Three of the patients listed in Table 7.1 showed reduplicative paramnesia in association with their Capgras delusion. Another showed reduplication of time. This is a rare reduplication syndrome that occurs following brain trauma (Weinstein, 1969, 1994) and has also been documented in the setting of dementia (Aziz & Warner, 2005): the patient believes that recent events, e.g. hospitalization for head injury or a tour of military duty, have occurred before, sometimes multiple times. Detailed descriptions of the phenomenon are hard to come by, but one such patient seen by the present author is described in Box 7.3.

Box 7.3 Reduplication of Time (From Tempest, M., Parthasarathi U., Walsh, C. and McKenna, P. J. Unpublished Case Report)

The patient was a university graduate in his twenties who underwent surgery for a pineal tumour. Two days afterwards he was noted to be confused; this improved rapidly, although his family noticed he remained slow and forgetful. Just under four weeks post-operatively he became abruptly distressed and began making statements about being in a 'time loop'.

On interview, the patient described having 'a constant feeling of déjà vu': if he read a book he would feel he had read it previously, but due to his poor memory he could not predict exactly how it would end. When he played backgammon he felt he had played the games before; when watching the long jump in the Olympic games he thought he knew how far each competitor would jump. He also had frequent periods where time went subjectively very slowly. These occurred up to ten times a day and during them it would feel as though up to several days had passed.

He went on to explain that the experience of déjà vu led him to wonder if he had already been through the current period of time before, and then to believe that he might be caught in a time loop. His degree of conviction in this belief fluctuated, but at times he claimed he was 90 per cent convinced that he was living through repeated cycles of time which lasted from days to as long as a month. He gave the example of going to sleep at on the 16th August and waking back up on 13th August. At the height of this state he expressed the idea that he would have to terminate these time loops by carrying out certain specific acts; one of these was committing suicide (he had a vague memory of committing suicide by different means in previous time cycles). He also entertained the possibility that what he was experiencing was imposed upon him by 'perpetrators', who were either aliens or people from the future. In relation to this, he half-recollected being on a table surrounded by human figures who were carrying out some form of procedure on him.

Structured interview using the PSE did not disclose any further psychotic symptoms, and he did not meet criteria for major depression. He was fully orientated and scored maximally on a general test of cognitive function, the MMSE. On neuropsychological testing there was evidence of mild to moderate memory impairment, affecting both recall and recognition. In contrast, executive function, picture naming, copy of a complex figure, and a test of object recognition were all normal. Investigations including a 24-hour EEG, were also normal. An MRI scan showed changes consistent with recent brain surgery, but was otherwise unremarkable.

After a few days, during which the patient was started on treatment with citalopram (an antidepressant), the experiences of déjà vu became less intrusive. His symptoms receded further over the next few weeks. His memory also improved over this period according to his family. Five months after surgery he was back at work and had full insight into his symptoms.

The Capgras syndrome is where the cognitive neuropsychology of delusions comes into its own. In 1990, Ellis and Young (the latter author is a leading authority on the psychology of face processing) proposed that the disorder might represent the mirror image of the neurological syndrome of prosopagnosia, an inability to recognize familiar faces that can occur after damage to parts of the occipital and temporal lobes. A notable characteristic of prosopagnosia is that, while the patients are often completely unable to identify photographs of famous people or family members, some of them show evidence of covert recognition. This can be demonstrated, for example, by the fact that changes in skin conductance occur when they are shown the face of a friend or relative (Bauer, 1984). This phenomenon is widely believed to reflect the existence of two separate routes for the processing of familiar face information: one underlies conscious recognition (and is sometimes referred to as the ventral route because its ultimate destination is part of the temporal lobe cortex), and the other gives rise to the emotional accompaniments of recognizing a familiar person (the so-called dorsal route that connects the visual cortex to the limbic system). If damage to the former route results in prosopagnosia, Ellis and Young (1990) argued, damage to the latter might well result in the kind of experience that lies at the heart of the Capgras syndrome:

> [P]atients with Capgras' syndrome seem to have an intact primary or ventral route to face recognition, but may have a disconnection along or damage within the secondary or dorsal route. This would mean that they receive a veridical image of the person they are looking at, which stimulates all the appropriate overt semantic data held about that person, but they lack another, possibly confirming, set of information which … may carry some sort of affective tone. When patients find themselves in such a conflict (that is, receiving some information which indicates the face in front of them belongs to X, but not receiving confirmation of this), they may adopt some sort of rationalization strategy in which the individual before them is deemed to be an imposter, a dummy, a robot, or whatever extant technology may suggest.

Ellis et al. (1997) found some support for this proposal in a study of five psychiatric patients with the Capgras delusion, who they compared with five psychiatric patients without the delusion and five healthy subjects. Diagnostic criteria were not employed but the Capgras patients and the psychiatric controls all had other psychotic symptoms. The healthy controls and the psychiatric controls both showed significantly larger skin conductance changes to a series of famous faces than to unfamiliar faces. This was not seen in the Capgras patients, where the response to both the familiar and unfamiliar faces was small. A neurological Capgras patient (Hirstein and Ramachandran's (1997) head injury patient in Table 7.1) was also found to show the same pattern of reduced skin conductance changes to photographs of both famous people and members of his family.

Compelling though it is, the mirror image prosopagnosia hypothesis of the Capgras syndrome faces a by now familiar problem. In the words of Hirstein and Ramachandran (1997): '[W]hy does the mere absence of this emotional arousal lead to such an extraordinarily far-fetched delusion? Why doesn't the patient just think, "I know that is my father but I no longer feel the warmth"?'. Worse still, neurological patients have been described (with damage to the ventromedial frontal cortex in all cases) who show lack of autonomic arousal to familiar faces, but do not have the Capgras syndrome (Tranel et al., 1995). After an in-depth consideration of this problem, Stone and Young (1997) concluded that an additional factor needed to be present. However, they were unable to come up with a clear answer to what this might be and ended up speculating, somewhat unsatisfactorily, that the brain injury that gives rise to the mirror image of prosopagnosia sometimes also produces an increase in general suspiciousness or a tendency to jump to conclusions.

Coltheart and co-workers were less easily put off. Over a period of approximately fifteen years they pursued various possibilities and slowly arrived at a theory of what the additional factor might be. Their initial position (Davies & Coltheart, 2000; Langdon & Coltheart, 2000) was that another cognitive system was damaged alongside the one producing the failure to react emotionally to familiar faces. The function of this second system was difficult to characterize precisely, but seemed to involve a failure 'to allow antecedent beliefs or stored knowledge to trump the deliverances of perceptual experience'. This could not be a general failure, however, because if it was, Capgras patients would also fail to doubt the evidence of their own senses in other circumstances – for example, they would not be able to accept that optical illusions were just a trick. If this was the case, Coltheart and co-workers pointed out, someone would probably have noticed.

A few years later, and now drawing on findings from anosognosia and confabulation, they (Coltheart, 2005; Coltheart et al., 2007) felt they were in a position to specify the putative belief evaluation process more precisely. It was, they proposed, a moment-to-moment, automatic process whereby predictions generated about what was going to happen were compared against what actually took place. When this system registered that a prediction was not confirmed – in this case, seeing one's wife and not experiencing the accompanying jolt of emotional recognition – it would trigger off a review of relevant knowledge: 'the unconscious system makes some kind of report to consciousness to instigate some intelligent conscious problem-solving behavior that will discover what's wrong with the database and how it should be repaired'. In patients with the Capgras syndrome, they proposed that either the initial registration of the untoward event or the later problem-solving behaviour, or both, failed to occur. Why this failure did not lead to generalized problems affecting all kinds of stray thoughts entering the patients' heads was still a problem, but Coltheart speculated that the repeated nature of the experience of emotional non-recognition might be important.

The most recent version of the theory (Turner & Coltheart, 2010; Coltheart et al., 2011) is explicitly an expansion of the strategic retrieval theory of memory. Coltheart and co-workers now argue that it is not just memory traces activated by synergistic ecphory that undergo checking for veridicality, but all information entering conscious awareness. This checking occurs in two stages, the first being an effortless, automatic process that endows incoming information with a feeling of rightness, and the second being a more labour-intensive thinking through of the implications of accepting the information as true. Of these two processes, Turner and Coltheart (2010) were attracted particularly to the former as the culprit in the Capgras delusion:

> Reasoning processes are usually thought of as conscious, and yet conscious reasoning seems not to be involved at all in many delusions and confabulations. More often, delusional and confabulatory ideas seen to enter consciousness fully formed with the patients unaware of any prior unusual experience. Certainly the rest of us who are not delusional or confabulatory are not aware of consciously considering and then rejecting the kinds of bizarre thoughts that delusional and confabulating patients espouse.

Turner and Coltheart (2010) also speculated on how such an automatic, preconscious checking system might work. One possibility involved novelty: it could be that experiences, memories and beliefs the person has previously been exposed to were automatically passed by the system, whereas new ones were tagged as requiring full conscious checking. Or perhaps the system was somehow able to detect whether the incoming information was associated with an appropriate amount of supporting knowledge, and triggered the full checking process if it was not. Or possibly what the system was sensitive to was conflicts, either between the different elements of the item of information or between all of it and the rest of the person's knowledge. Finally, they (Turner and Coltheart, 2010) raised the possibility that the process might not actually consist of attaching a feeling of rightness to items of information that passed the first stage of checking, but instead of attachment of a 'feeling of doubt' to those that did not. This would have the advantage of being less resource demanding.

Conclusion: Is the Two Factor Theory Viable and If So What Does It Mean?

The occurrence of phenomena in neurological disease that are similar to (and in the case of the Capgras syndrome identical to) delusions provides an unprecedented opportunity to gain new insights into the underlying cognitive and brain mechanisms of the symptom. Or at least it should do: the less than desirable result of the work in this area has been a lot of theorizing but few hard facts. Nevertheless, judging the two factor theory on its own, largely theoretical merits, there seem to be two important questions facing it. The first is how credible the concept of a brain system dedicated to a process of fact checking is. The second is whether malfunction in such a system can really be understood in the way it is almost always construed, as a deficit.

On the face of it, what the two factor theory proposes – that there is a system in the brain which continuously checks all information entering conscious awareness for compatibility with all the rest of the individual's knowledge, this being achieved effortlessly and without any awareness that it is taking place – is far from intuitive. It could, however, be argued that this is no more than what the facts demand. If confabulation, and monothematic forms of the Capgras syndrome (and possibly also anosognosia for hemiplegia) are ever going to be explained, it seems unavoidable that some process along these lines will have to be invoked; nothing simpler will suffice. It is almost a case of what Sherlock Holmes described as when the impossible has been eliminated whatever remains, however improbable, must be the truth.

As regards the nature of the second factor, if it involves attribution of feeling of rightness, then logically it cannot be a deficit. The problem is not that feeling of rightness fails to be applied to information entering conscious awareness; rather, it gets attached when it ought not to be – to erroneous ecphorized memories in confabulation and to an explanation of an experience that ought immediately be rejected in the case of the Capgras syndrome. A deficit conceptualization can only be reinstated if, as Turner and Coltheart (2010) raised as a possibility, what gets attached to information is not a feeling of rightness when it passes preliminary checks, but instead a feeling of doubt when it does not. However, this idea is speculative and swims against the tide of current neurological thinking.

The second factor could also be a deficit if it occurred not at the stage of assigning feeling of rightness but during the later subsequent deliberate checking for consistency with the rest of the person's knowledge. However, as Turner and Coltheart (2010) noted, this would rob the delusion of its quality of arising fully formed with no contribution of conscious reasoning – in short, of being unmediated.

If the second factor is not a deficit, what could it be? The answer to this question may lie in the points made in Chapter 5, that brain damage does not always result in deficits, and that dysfunctions in complicated cognitive systems can take a rich variety of forms. It is not difficult to envisage a situation where impaired function in one brain system or cognitive module allows the function of another to go unchecked. Or perhaps the second system continues to function more or less normally but without some critical part of its input that allows it to automatically correct its output or perform with the right degree of flexibility.

Perhaps the most important question facing monothematic delusions is whether they have any significance for delusions as a whole. One obvious answer here is that they might underlie the phenomenon of delusional explanations. As Coltheart (2005) has pointed out, the first factor, which gives rise to the experience the delusion is based on, is different in the different forms of delusion-like phenomenon seen in neurological disease, but the second factor is the same in all cases. If so, Frith's explanation of delusions of control in schizophrenia in terms of a failure of efference copy when making a movement could easily provide a further example, as could the idea that the Cotard syndrome is an elaboration of the experience of depersonalization. In principle, there seems to be no reason why the same explanation could not also applied to schizophrenic patients who explain their auditory hallucinations as being due a microchip in their heads, or to depressed patients whose depressive cognitions are converted into delusions of guilt, etc. Could it be that the explanatory power of the second factor goes further still, and forms a unifying basis for all propositional delusions? This is a possibility that is raised in the final chapter of this book.

The Salience Theory of Delusions

Theoretical approaches to delusions often seem to have a curiously half-hearted quality. No one has ever bothered to test Maher's theory. Theory of mind abnormality and probabilistic reasoning bias have both run into significant experimental difficulties, and there has been little enthusiasm for addressing them. Important features of delusions such as their impossibility and imperviousness to reason are generally given only token consideration, and in most cases referential delusions are ignored altogether.

Such criticisms do not apply to a further approach to delusions, Kapur's (2003) salience theory. This has been so influential that it recently led to a serious attempt to rename schizophrenia as salience dysregulation disorder (van Os, 2009) – despite the fact that it has only very limited power to explain any other class of symptom besides delusions. Its power derives partly from the fact that it provides an intuitive explanation of what this book collectively refers to as referential delusions. Another source of strength is the central role it accords to dopamine which, despite its many setbacks, is still an important player in schizophrenia research. Nor does it hurt that the principal means of testing the theory involves stepping into the glamorous if not always easily understandable world of functional brain imaging.

Clearly, such an important theory demands detailed and critical consideration, to make sure that its claims hold up theoretically and to examine how far they are supported by evidence. There is also another reason for engaging in such an exercise. This is that the theory only tells half the story. In particular, it will be argued that, while the salience theory's explanation of referential delusions is compelling, what it says about propositional delusions is no more substantial than in any other theory of delusions. Another aim of this chapter, therefore, will be to explore what can be done to repair this weakness. As it turns out, efforts in this direction go back to well before the salience theory appeared on the scene and continue right up to the present time.

Introducing the Salience Theory

The salience theory starts with an assumption. This is that the dopamine hypothesis of schizophrenia is correct, specifically that a functional excess of the neurotransmitter underlies the positive symptoms of the disorder. If this is so, then it follows that these symptoms should be understandable in terms of what is known about the normal function of dopamine. For Kapur (2003), this function was the way in which it acts to assign motivational and reinforcing value to stimuli that are associated with reward (see Chapter 6). Pathologically increased dopamine transmission would then lead to a release of dopamine outside the proper context, which in turn would cause neutral stimuli to inappropriately acquire significance for behaviour, or as Kapur termed it, aberrant salience.

The subjective correlate of saliences being created when there ought not to be any might be that the individual would start to wrongly experience neutral events as important. Such a hypothetical state, Kapur (2003) noted, matched closely with the descriptions that schizophrenic patients gave of the earliest stages of their illness, as recorded in a spate of studies carried out in the 1960s. These included statements such as: 'I developed a greater awareness of ... My senses were sharpened. I became fascinated by the little insignificant things around me,' and 'Sights and sounds possessed a keenness that he had never experienced before' (Bowers & Freedman, 1966); 'It was as if parts of my brain awoke, which had been dormant' (McDonald, 1960); or 'My senses seemed alive ... Things seemed clearcut, I noticed things I had never noticed before' (Bowers, 1968). Related to this there might also be a feeling that the world was changing in a puzzling way that required explanation. This was also evident in the patients' accounts, for example, 'I felt that there was some overwhelming significance in this' (McDonald, 1960), and 'I felt like I was putting a piece of the puzzle together' (Bowers, 1968).

Delusions – by which Kapur (2003) meant propositional delusions in the terminology of this book – were proposed to be the result of the individual's effort to make sense of the experience of aberrant salience as it was repeated over days, months or years:

> Delusions in this framework are a 'top-down' cognitive explanation that the individual imposes on these experiences of aberrant salience in an effort to make sense of them. Since delusions are constructed by the individual, they are imbued with the psychodynamic themes relevant to the individual and are embedded in the cultural context of the individual. This explains how the same neurochemical dysregulation leads to variable phenomenological expression: a patient in Africa struggling to make sense of aberrant saliences is much more likely to accord them to the evil ministrations of a shaman, while the one living in Toronto is more likely to see them as the machinations of the Royal Canadian Mounted Police.

Kapur (2003) did not rule out the possibility that additional factors might contribute to the process whereby fully formed delusions developed out of the initially amorphous experience of aberrant salience. These could include a jumping to conclusions cognitive style and poorly developed theory of mind skills, and perhaps aspects of the patient's personality as well.

Kapur (2003) considered that delusions of reference and misinterpretation also arose as part of the attempt at explanation. This drove the patient to search for further confirmatory evidence within the evolving delusional framework, 'in the glances of strangers, in the headlines of newspapers, and in the lapel pins of newscasters'.

This then is the theory. It is not difficult to see why it has become so influential: it provides, perhaps for the first time in the history of schizophrenia research, a simple and intellectually satisfying link between a symptom of the disorder and an underlying biological brain disturbance. If dopamine causes neutral stimuli in the environment to acquire significance – and following the work of Schultz (1998) described in Chapter 6, there seems no doubt that it does – then it seems highly probable that a dopamine excess will give rise to a state which resembles delusional mood. Although not explicitly part of Kapur's theory, there does not seem to be any particular difficulty extending the same concept to encompass all other types of delusion whose central phenomenological feature is an abnormal feeling of significance.

Where the theory fares less well is in its explanation of propositional delusions. The main proposal offered here is that this class of delusions represents an attempt by the individual to make sense of the experience of aberrant salience. As such, this part of the theory is not obviously an advance over what Maher (1974) proposed 40 years ago (see Chapter 5). To be sure, the salience theory avoids one problem Maher ran into, that of having to invoke a 'free-floating feeling of significance' to explain how delusions arise when there are no accompanying perceptual abnormalities. On the other hand, in exactly the same way as Maher's approach, the theory struggles to explain several phenomenological features of propositional delusions, especially the fact that they tend to the bizarre and fantastic.

Finally, and perhaps most importantly, the salience theory makes the prediction that propositional delusions will always be preceded by delusional mood and/or other referential delusions. This is something that, as Chapters 1 and 3 make clear, is by no means always the case in practice.

Can the Salience Theory Be Extended to Explain Propositional Delusions?

Before Kapur introduced the salience theory in 2003, a few other authors had tried to link dopamine to delusions. One of these was Beninger (1983) who, in the course of a review of the role of dopamine in behaviour, suggested that an overstimulation of dopamine receptors might have the consequence that schizophrenic patients would lose their ability to ignore irrelevant stimuli, and that paranoia or delusions of grandeur could represent cognitive elaborations of the apparent meaningfulness of these stimuli. The present author (McKenna, 1987, 1991) proposed something quite similar as one part of an attempt to link dopamine to a wide range of schizophrenic symptoms.

But it was another author who came up with the first concrete proposal for how a hyper-dopaminergic state might give rise to propositional delusions. Miller (1984) argued that the associative processes of learning, i.e. the formation of links between stimuli and stimuli (classical or Pavlovian conditioning) and between stimuli and responses (instrumental learning), might also take place at a higher level, leading to the formation of cognitive associations. If so, he speculated, the role of dopamine would in effect be to set the threshold for inductive inference:

> For any step of inductive inference there must be a threshold, or set point, comparable in some ways to a criterion of significance in a statistical argument. Below this threshold associational links are rejected as coincidental. Above the threshold they are 'above chance', and, therefore, accepted as real.

A functional increase in dopamine would lower this set point, causing a 'hyperactivity of inductive inference'. This would lead to more cognitive associations than normal being formed, many of which would be spurious. To the extent that these associative links could be equated with conceptual thinking, the result would be propositional delusions.

The idea of dopamine exerting effects on higher cognitive function was controversial enough, and Miller's proposal that it somehow acted to set the threshold for inductive inference was a leap in the dark. But as it happened, his idea resonated with those in a book that had just been published to considerable acclaim (one reviewer compared it to Newton's *Principia Mathematica*), which argued that animals routinely do something very similar to making inductive inferences. This was Gray's (1981) theory of hippocampal (or as he preferred to call it, septo-hippocampal) function, and it was destined to play a significant role in the subsequent evolution of thinking about the role of dopamine in delusions.

Gray's (1981) theory was a highly complicated tour de force that integrated an enormous number of animal behavioural findings on the hippocampus and septal area with almost as much neuroanatomy and neurophysiology. However, at its core the proposal was simple: the hippocampus acts as a comparator, matching, on a moment-to-moment basis, 'actual', i.e. the currently perceived state of the world, with 'expected', or predictions about what ought to be experienced after the animal performs the next step in the sequence of motor acts it is carrying out. Gray noted that the hippocampus was well equipped to receive information about the actual state of the world via its major afferent pathway from the entorhinal cortex; this was known to be a destination for highly analysed sensory information in all modalities. He proposed that the predictive function was accomplished by means of the classical Papez circuit running from the hippocampus to the cingulate cortex (and also the prefrontal cortex in primates) via the mammillary bodies and the thalamus, before projecting back to the entorhinal cortex.

The main way in which the system exerted an effect on behaviour was through what Gray (1981) called behavioural inhibition – a sudden interruption of the sequence of motor responses currently being executed when a mismatch between actual and expected was detected. How the hippocampus managed to gain access to motor systems to produce behavioural inhibition was something of a mystery at the time his book was published. However, a year later an efferent projection from the subiculum (the main output area of the hippocampus) to the ventral striatum was described (Kelley & Domesick, 1982), something that filled the role perfectly.

The septo-hippocampal system could also operate in a 'just checking' mode, when observed matched with expected. In this case the sequence of motor responses being elaborated was allowed to proceed without interruption. When the animal found itself in a new environment, where no predictions could be made, the system fell into yet another, 'exploratory' mode (see Box 8.1).

Box 8.1 Gray's Proposed Modes of Septo-hippocampal Function (Gray, 1981)

Scenario 1: Exposure to a Novel Environment

The animal is in a totally new environment. Under these conditions there can be no predictions for the comparator to match against current experience. It follows that the only task the septo-hippocampal system can perform is gathering information that will make subsequent prediction possible. Information about the novel events is passed on for storage elsewhere.

Scenario 2: Just Checking

There exists a set of expectations which continue to be verified by current sensory input. Under these conditions the system exercises no control over behaviour.

Scenario 3: Mismatch

The comparator detects a mismatch between expected and actual events. In this situation the septo-hippocampal system assumes control over behaviour. Major features of this mode of operation include the active inhibition of motor behaviour and the institution of information-gathering strategies with the aim of resolving the discrepancy. These two together – analysis and exploration – constitute a process analogous to hypothesis generation and testing. Other consequences include tagging the motor programme as 'faulty, needs checking', and executing it more cautiously on future occasions.

Scenario 4: Disengagement
After the discrepancy has been resolved behavioural control passes back to other systems which may, however, now receive updated information as a result of the activities of the septo-hippocampal system.

Two other features of Gray's (1981) theory were also important. One was that information about matches and mismatches was proposed to be passed on to other brain regions where it was used to modify future predictions about what was to be expected in that particular environment (and also to form new predictions in the case of a novel environment). The other was that two modulatory neurotransmitters, noradrenalin and serotonin, which were at the time known to innervate the hippocampus, acted to label stimuli that were novel or associated with aversive events as 'important, check carefully', and to bias the system towards behavioural inhibition. In fact, a large part of the raison d'être of Gray's theory was for him to be able to argue that dysfunction in one or both of these transmitters systems would lead to overly frequent behavioural inhibition, which in turn formed the basis of anxiety disorders. He also speculated that the environmental checking that was instituted after behavioural inhibition took place might serve as a model for obsessive-compulsive disorder.

It seemed only a matter of time before the theory would also be applied to schizophrenia, and ten years later Gray and several co-workers (Gray et al., 1991) duly did so. Their main innovation was to add dopamine, which by now was by now also known to innervate the hippocampus, to the model of septo-hippocampal function. Unlike noradrenalin and serotonin, this neurotransmitter was proposed to operate in the system's 'just checking' mode, where it acted to facilitate the transition from one step in a motor programme to the next when no conflict between observed and expected was detected. Excess dopamine, Gray et al. (1991) argued, would result in a special kind of disorder in motor programming whereby one or more responses became inappropriately dominant. (Although the authors said nothing about reduced dopamine in their 1991 article, an interesting aside is that the consequences of this would presumably be something not dissimilar to the akinesia and bradykinesia of Parkinsonism.)

Motor responses becoming inappropriately dominant is a long way from delusions, and Gray et al.'s (1991) main suggestion with respect to these and other psychotic symptoms was that the disturbance caused by a dopamine excess might also extend to the programming of selective attention. More broadly, they also felt that their proposal was consistent with a suggestion for understanding positive psychotic symptoms that had been made a few years earlier by one of the authors of the article (Helmsley, 1987), that they reflected a 'a weakening of the influence of stored memories or regularities of previous input on current perception'. If nothing else, this proposal has the dubious distinction of being one of the least testable hypotheses ever formulated in schizophrenia research.

Years later, after the publication of Kapur's salience theory, Gray (2004) wrote a letter claiming that he and his co-authors, in their 1991 article, had themselves proposed that aberrant salience would be a further consequence of a dopamine excess affecting the septo-hippocampal system. As far as the present author can tell, there is no statement to this effect in the article. Gray (1998), however, did note this possibility in a subsequent paper.

Today, Gray's theory languishes in obscurity, eclipsed by a rival theory that he did his best to disparage in his 1981 book, O'Keefe and Nadel's (1978) cognitive map proposal (which ultimately won one of its authors the Nobel Prize). Nevertheless, the concept of a brain system that compares actual and expected and whose dysfunction gives rise to delusions lives on in the work of a loosely knit group of researchers which includes but is not limited to Corlett, Fletcher, Friston and Frith (e.g. Fletcher & Frith, 2009; Corlett et al., 2009; Corlett et al., 2010b; Adams et al., 2013). For these authors, forming predictions is a general mode of brain function, which is carried out based on Bayesian statistical principles and which underlies not only learning but also perception and in all probability other cognitive processes as well. Equally important is prediction error, to which this process is inextricably linked: predictive models form the basis for the generation of prediction errors, and prediction errors in turn modify the predictive model. At times the theory is almost explicitly Grayian in tone: Corlett et al. (2010b) suggested that when an organism experiences an event that violates predictions, an orienting system is activated which enables the acquisition of new data for a new predictive model. In contrast, when the event matches what is predicted, the current predictive model of the world is strengthened.

With respect to the formation of delusions, Corlett et al. (2010b) agreed with Kapur (2003) that:

> during the earliest phases of delusion formation aberrant novelty, salience or prediction error signals drive attention toward redundant or irrelevant environmental cues, the world seems to have changed, it feels strange and sinister…

But now, the occurrence of erroneous prediction errors also leads to a modification of the predictive model of the relevant aspect of the world:

> … such signals and experiences provide an impetus for new learning which updates the world model inappropriately, manifest as a delusion.

To which Fletcher and Frith (2009) added that the model of the world can never be successful because it can never eliminate the prediction error. The rogue signal persists however many attempts are made to accommodate it, and so the predictive model deviates more and more from reality.

With this, via a circuitous route involving thresholds for inductive inference and a defunct theory of hippocampal function, the salience theory has arrived at its current state of the art. It now has the benefit not only of an intuitive account of referential delusions, but also something that seems close to a credible explanation of propositional delusions. This qualification 'close to' needs to be appended, because the theory still predicts that propositional delusions will always be preceded by delusional mood and/or referential delusions. It also depends on there being a mechanism whereby dopamine (or possibly some other neurotransmitter) directly influences cognition. As far as the present author is aware, there is as yet no evidence for such a proposal.

Testing the Salience Theory

Increased Dopamine in Schizophrenia

With its simple and intuitive explanation of referential delusions and the strong hints it may be sooner or later also be able to provide an account of propositional delusions, the salience theory certainly talks a good game. But as with any other theory, the only thing that ultimately counts is whether it can gain experimental support. One relevant line of experimental evidence already exists in the form of the dopamine hypothesis of schizophrenia itself – if this were proved to be correct, it would be a good first step towards the salience theory also being correct, particularly since dopamine appears to have a particular role in positive symptoms.

Unfortunately, whether the dopamine hypothesis is right or wrong has become something of an eternal question, whose definitive proof one way or the other always seems just out of reach. The proposal was first intensively investigated following the discovery, made more or less simultaneously by three different groups of investigators, that post-synaptic dopamine D2 receptor numbers in the basal ganglia were increased in the post-mortem brains of schizophrenic patients (see Seeman, 1987). It was quickly realized that this finding did not in itself constitute proof of anything, because almost all the patients in these studies had been treated with antipsychotic drugs in life, and antipsychotic treatment itself can cause D2 receptor numbers to increase (as a compensatory response to their blockade by these drugs). What was needed were studies examining D2 receptor numbers in never-treated schizophrenic patients. Although challenging, this goal was achieved some years later by combining functional imaging with use of a tracer that attached to D2 receptors (i.e. a radioactively labelled antipsychotic) in living patients who had received little or no previous drug treatment. The first study (Wong et al., 1986), carried out on a group of chronic schizophrenic patients who for one reason or another had never been given drug treatment, found an approximate doubling of basal ganglia D2 receptor numbers compared to healthy controls. The second (Farde et al., 1990), carried out on drug naïve first-episode patients, found no difference. For a time the fate of this version of the dopamine hypothesis hung in the balance, but eventually a series of further studies (Martinot et al., 1990; Hietala et al., 1994; Pilowsky et al., 1994) all supported the negative finding of Farde et al. (1990).

The second wave of studies took a different tack and tested the hypothesis that synaptic release of dopamine, as provoked by amphetamine, is increased in schizophrenic patients. Three studies, two by the same investigators (Laruelle et al., 1996; Abi-Dargham et al., 1998) and one by an independent group (Breier et al., 1997) all had positive findings. These studies were carried out in drug-free patients; however, only a minority of them were drug-naïve. Is it possible that the previous antipsychotic treatment in the majority of patients could have caused an increase in amphetamine-stimulated dopamine release? The answer appears to be yes: the technique used for measuring dopamine release in these studies depended on the displacement of radioactively labelled ligand from post-synaptic D2 receptors. As Laurelle et al. (1999) acknowledged, this meant that the differences found could conceivably have been due to increased dopamine binding to these receptors, caused by the patients' previous treatment, rather than by increased amphetamine-stimulated dopamine release per se. The authors of these studies had forgotten a basic principle of schizophrenia research: in order to convince sceptics (not to mention the many who are constitutionally opposed to any biological theory of the disorder), it is necessary to demonstrate that any alleged brain abnormality is present beyond a shadow of a doubt.

The third and current wave of studies was ushered in by a study that examined the dopamine hypothesis from yet another angle, of whether there is increased production of the neurotransmitter in schizophrenic patients. This study avoided the problem of prior antipsychotic treatment by adopting a strategy of examining patients who had prodromal symptoms of schizophrenia rather than the disorder itself. Howes et al. (2009) compared 24 patients with the so-called at-risk mental state and 12 matched healthy controls. The patients all showed evidence of attenuated psychotic symptoms and four had previously experienced brief, self-limiting episodes of psychosis. Only one had received treatment with antipsychotics and this was omitted for 24 hours before scanning. All subjects underwent functional imaging using a radioactively labelled form of the dopamine precursor, l-DOPA, and levels of radioactivity in the striatum in the two groups was compared under blind conditions.

The prodromal patients showed a 6.3 per cent increase in l-DOPA uptake compared to the controls in the whole striatal region, a significant difference. When the striatum was divided up into 'motor', 'associative' and 'limbic' subregions (the last corresponding to the ventral striatum), the elevation was found to be restricted to the associative sector. A small group of seven patients with schizophrenia (three drug-free, four treated) also showed a similar increase in l-DOPA uptake.

Howes and co-workers' subsequent studies have had mixed fortunes. The original finding was replicated in a second cohort of 26 high-risk subjects and 20 healthy controls (Egerton et al., 2013). The findings for both groups combined are shown in Figure 8.1. In a three-year follow-up of some of the members of both cohorts (Howes et al., 2011a), it was found that the nine who went on to develop full-blown psychosis (schizophrenia in four, schizophreniform psychosis in one and mania with psychotic symptoms in one) had significantly higher baseline levels of striatal dopamine uptake than those who did not. However, this result was only achieved after six high-risk individuals were removed from the analysis on the rather shaky grounds that they also had a diagnosis of schizotypal personality disorder. When Howes et al. (2011b) directly compared l-DOPA uptake before and after the onset of psychosis in eight patients, there was no significant increase in the striatum as a whole, nor in the limbic or associative sectors; however, a significant increase was seen in the sensorimotor sector. A summary of these latter findings is also shown in Figure 8.1.

Reward-Associated Ventral Striatal Activation in Psychosis

Whether the dopamine hypothesis of schizophrenia can be considered proved as a result of the last two waves of investigation is undecided – attitudes currently range from self-satisfied complacency to world-weary cynicism – but even if it is, this does not automatically mean that the salience theory is also correct To establish this, and once again convince what will no doubt be a legion of sceptics, some way needs to be found to show that patients with delusions attribute salience abnormally.

Fortunately, such a way exists. By the end of the 1990s, functional imaging studies had demonstrated that the experience of reward, ranging from receiving a small amount of fruit juice and seeing attractive faces at one end of the spectrum, to viewing erotic videos and being administered cocaine at the other, produced a pattern of activation in the brain (McClure et al., 2004). The regions activated were broadly similar to those known to be involved in reward in animals, including the ventral striatum, the amygdala and an area encompassing the orbitofrontal and ventromedial prefrontal cortex. Then Knutson and co-workers (Knutson et al., 2000, 2001a, 2001b) devised a functional magnetic resonance imaging (fMRI) paradigm involving one of the most reliable, powerful and easy to manipulate rewards of all, money.

A representation of their paradigm, the monetary incentive delay (MID) task is shown in Figure 8.2. Subjects have to perform a reaction time task (pressing a button when they see a white square before it disappears) whose difficulty is individually adjusted during a

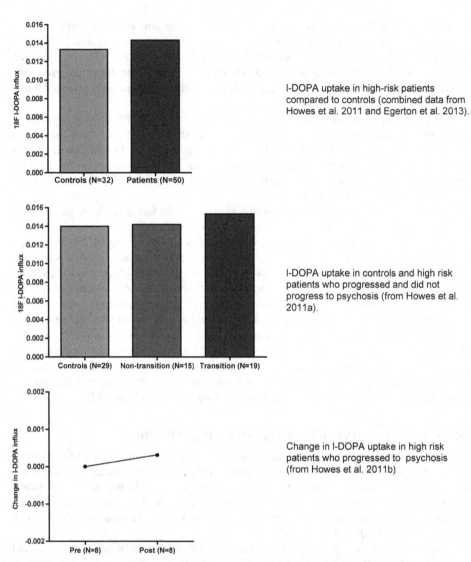

I-DOPA uptake in high-risk patients compared to controls (combined data from Howes et al. 2011 and Egerton et al. 2013).

I-DOPA uptake in controls and high risk patients who progressed and did not progress to psychosis (from Howes et al. 2011a).

Change in I-DOPA uptake in high risk patients who progressed to psychosis (from Howes et al. 2011b)

Figure 8.1 Howes and co-workers' studies of dopamine synthesis in patients with the at-risk mental state. *Source*: From Egerton, A., et al., 2013. Presynaptic striatal dopamine dysfunction in people at ultra-high risk for psychosis: findings in a second cohort. *Biological Psychiatry*, 74, 106–112; Howes, O. D., et al., 2011a. Dopamine synthesis capacity before onset of psychosis: a prospective [18F]-DOPA PET imaging study. *American Journal of Psychiatry*, 168, 1311–1317, reproduced with permission; Howes, O., et al., 2011b. Progressive increase in striatal dopamine synthesis capacity as patients develop psychosis: a PET study. *Molecular Psychiatry*, 16, 885–886.

training phase so that they are successful approximately two-thirds of the time. On some trials, the task is preceded by a cue, for example a circle, which signals that they will win a certain amount of money if they perform the reaction time task successfully. Other trials are preceded by a different cue, for example a triangle, which indicates that successful performance will have no monetary consequences. Feedback about whether they have won

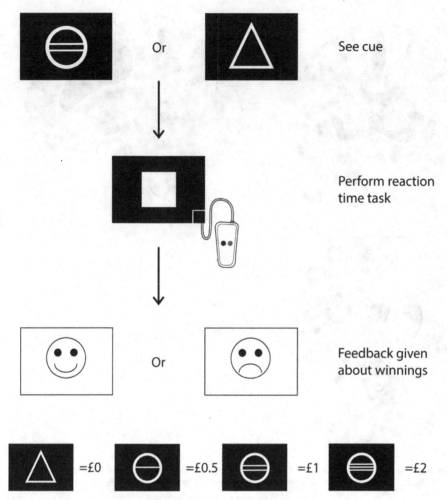

Or   See cue

Perform reaction time task

Or   Feedback given about winnings

=£0   =£0.5   =£1   =£2

Figure 8.2 The monetary incentive delay (MID) task.

is presented immediately after the response is made. Activation in response to the reward signalling cue compared to the neutral cue provides a measure of the extent to which different brain regions respond to salience.

In many versions of the task the amount of money that can be won on a particular trial varies, and this is indicated, for example by the number of bars superimposed on the cue. There are many other variations of the task – in some, rather than being pretrained, the subjects have to learn the predictive values of the cues by trial and error while being scanned, and in others there is no interpolated reaction time task. These and other modifications make it possible to also measure reward prediction error.

In their first study, Knutson et al. (2000) examined activations in a number of predetermined regions of interest (ROIs): the nucleus accumbens, the caudate nucleus, the putamen, the thalamus, the anterior cingulate cortex and the medial frontal cortex. Twelve healthy

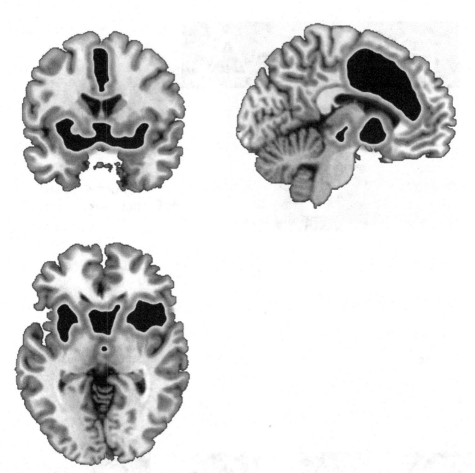

Figure 8.3 Meta-analysis of 25 voxel-based fMRI studies of reward anticipation. Studies included those which used the MID task, as well as other tasks where there the reward was monetary, and where the analysis covered the whole brain.
Source: Jauhar, S., Solanes, A., McKenna, P. J., & Radua, J., unpublished data.

subjects were found to show significant cue-related activation in the caudate nucleus and putamen and the medial prefrontal cortex, though not in the nucleus accumbens. In later studies (e.g. Knutson et al., 2001a, 2001b, 2005; Bjork et al., 2004) they replaced ROI analysis with the so-called whole-brain approach which compares the activity of every voxel in the brain (or a proportion of it) in the two conditions, and generates a map of significant differences. These studies additionally documented activation in the ventral striatum.

Jauhar et al. (unpublished) meta-analysed these and other voxel-based fMRI studies of monetary reward anticipation. The findings are shown in Figure 8.3. There was significant activation in large areas of the basal ganglia, including both its dorsal and ventral sectors. This finding tends to support Schultz's (1998) findings in monkeys described in Chapter 6, that dopaminergic neurons coding reward prediction error are distributed throughout the

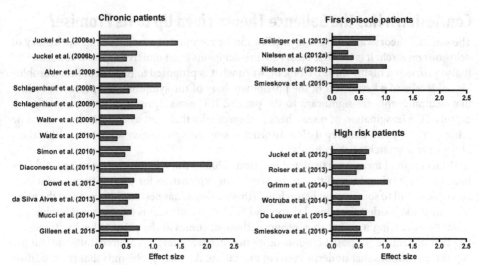

Figure 8.4 Radua et al.'s meta-analysis of fMRI studies examining ventral striatal activation in response to anticipation of monetary reward in schizophrenia, first episode psychosis and those at clinical or genetic high risk. Upper and lower bars in each study are for the left and right ventral striatum.
Source: From Radua, J., et al., 2015. Ventral striatal activation during reward processing in psychosis: a neurofunctional meta-analysis. *JAMA Psychiatry*, 72, 1243–1251; raw data kindly provided by Quim Radua.

striatum, not just its ventral striatal sector. A large and well-defined cortical area encompassing the anterior and middle cingulate cortex and other parts of the medial frontal was also activated, again in line with animal studies. The third main area that was activated was the bilateral insula, a cortical region whose function remains uncertain. Finally, activation was seen in the midbrain, reasonably close to but not actually involving its dopaminergic regions.

The way was now clear to directly test the hypothesis that there is aberrant salience in schizophrenia, and to determine whether it is associated with presence of delusions. Over 20 such studies have been carried out so far. These have examined medicated patients with schizophrenia, as well as samples of first-episode patients, some of whom were drug free or drug naïve, and also high-risk subjects. Radua et al. (2015) meta-analysed 23 such studies which employed an ROI placed in the ventral striatum. The pooled effect size was 0.50 for the left nucleus accumbens (in the medium range) and 0.70 on the right (in the medium to large range). As shown in Figure 8.4, a notable feature is that the effect, although individually variable, is in the same direction in all studies. The bad news is that the direction is the wrong one: patients with schizophrenia, first-episode psychosis and the at-risk mental state show reduced ventral stwriatal activation in response to reward-predicting stimuli, rather than the increased activation that the salience theory requires.

Eight studies in Radua et al.'s (2015) meta-analysis used measures of reward prediction error rather than just measuring the difference in activation between reward-predicting and neutral cues. The pooled findings were again in the direction of this being lower in patients than controls. Six studies examined the relationship between ventral striatal activation and positive symptoms. No significant association was found, although the authors cautioned that this result might not be reliable due to the small number of studies and also the heterogeneity among them.

Conclusions: Has the Salience Theory Lived Up to Its Promise?

The salience theory can with some justification be regarded as a milestone in the history of delusions research. It is the first theory to link delusions to an underlying brain abnormality. It also provides a highly intuitive link between what is proposed to happen at the neurobiological level and a key aspect of the phenomenology of the symptom, the pervasive feeling that neutral events are significant to the patient. It is not surprising, therefore, that it has captured the imagination of researchers (although why this went as far as trying to rename schizophrenia as salience regulation disorder is something that may leave future historians of psychiatry scratching their heads).

In its original form, as articulated by Kapur (2003), the salience theory had an Achilles heel, in that it offered very little in the way of an explanation for propositional delusions. Since then (and to some extent beforehand) this weakness has been recognized and the work of authors like Corlett, Fletcher, Friston and Frith currently seems to go a considerable way towards remedying it. What they propose, though, comes at the price of having to postulate that dopamine (or possibly some other neurotransmitter) has a direct influence on the cognitive processes that underlie concept formation. Another problem is that the modified theory still on the face of it predicts that propositional delusions will always be preceded by delusional mood.

At the experimental level, is aberrant salience an example of a beautiful theory destroyed by an ugly fact? At first sight it certainly looks that way, with what must be one of the most consistent findings in the history of schizophrenia research indicating that patients with schizophrenia show reduced rather than the predicted increased reward cue-related ventral striatal activity. However, unlike a finding of no change, this leaves the theory with some room for manoeuvre. It could be, for example, that salience attribution tends to be generally reduced in schizophrenia, perhaps related to negative symptoms, and this masks an increase in patients with delusions and other active psychotic symptoms. This is not a particularly strong position to take, given that Radua et al.'s (2015) meta-analysis revealed no hint of a correlation between ventral striatal activation and positive symptoms. Or it could be that simply comparing activations to reward-associated stimuli between patients and controls is the wrong approach to take, and reward prediction error is what needs to be measured. Once again, however, there is little comfort for this view in Radua et al.'s (2015) meta-analysis.

A third, more subtle argument is that reduced activation to reward predicting stimuli in psychosis is actually what would be expected to be seen. If the abnormality underlying delusions is pathologically increased attribution of salience to neutral stimuli, and assuming that attribution of salience to reward associated stimuli continues to occur normally, then subtracting the former from the latter, as is done in fMRI studies, would reveal reduced activation. A hint – no more than this – that something like along these lines may be going on comes from a study by Murray et al. (2008). They compared 13 mostly treated first-episode patients (11 of whom later went on to be given a diagnosis of schizophrenia) and 12 matched healthy controls on a monetary reward task where there was no interpolated reaction time task and in which the participants learnt the cue-reward association while they were being scanned. A whole-brain, voxel based comparison between the patients and controls revealed reduced activation in the patients in the midbrain, the ventral pallidum, the putamen, the hippocampus, the insula, the cingulate cortex, and the medial frontal and orbitofrontal cortex, among other areas; there were no differences between the groups in the ventral striatum (although these were found in a subsequent ROI analysis). However, the authors also noted that the difference in midbrain activations between the two groups was driven by a combination of attenuated response to reward prediction error in the patients together with an augmented response to neutral prediction error.

What a Theory of Delusions Might Look Like

After subjecting delusions to detailed scrutiny from the both clinical and research points of view, some questions about the former seem to be reasonably well answered. It may never be possible to define delusions in a way that avoids contradictions, but capturing their essential qualities may be less of a problem than generally thought. Besides delusions another important type of abnormal belief exists, the overvalued idea. Recognition of this form of psychopathology may have the potential to resolve some of the classification difficulties surrounding delusional disorder, especially those relating to its somatic subtype. Delusional disorder itself emerges as a bona fide clinical syndrome, but the evidence that a minority of cases evolve into schizophrenia and that there is also an association with affective disorder means that its nosology is quite unusual. The evidence that delusions are on a continuum with non-delusional beliefs is not as strong as van Os and his followers would like to believe – the only area where this appears to be unequivocally true is in major affective disorder, and even then it is not at all clear that the mild end of the continuum extends into the healthy population.

This leaves the central conundrum of the underlying nature of delusions. It was always going to be too much to hope that that the different approaches explored in the later chapters of this book would build progressively to a comprehensive theory. Nevertheless, it is striking how often the same ideas crop up again and again in different ways. One way to try and organize these apparent points of contact is by using a framework suggested by Fletcher and Frith (2009) in one of the articles cited in the last chapter. They argue that a successful explanation of psychotic symptoms needs to work at three levels: it must identify the abnormal process or processes occurring at the neurobiological level. It must then link these with abnormalities that are present at the psychological level. Finally, it must take into account the experience of the symptom concerned, by which they seem to mean that the explanation offered should be consistent with its phenomenological characteristics.

In the case of delusions, there are two major themes that recur across these levels. One of these is duality, the idea of the operation of two different processes. The other relates to the fact that delusions are by and large personal, i.e. centred on the individual him- or herself. A further issue that may or may not turn out to be addressable within the Fletcher and Frith framework concerns the nature of the relationship between referential and propositional delusions, especially the fact that theories often propose that propositional delusions grow out of referentialial delusions, whereas this is by no means always the case in clinical practice.

The Duality at the Heart of Delusions

Phenomenology, as Jones et al. (2003) observed in a previously referenced debate about the nature of delusions, is a discipline that seems to have fallen off the psychiatric syllabus in recent years. Before it did so, however, it provoked a dispute about the essential nature of the symptom. For Jaspers (1959), all delusions were characterized by changed awareness of meaning, which underwent a radical transformation to become immediate and intrusive. Schneider (1949), in contrast, argued that abnormal significance only properly applied to referential delusions (delusional perceptions in his terminology), and that propositional delusions (his delusional ideas and delusional intuitions) lacked this quality. For better or worse, this book has sided with Schneider and takes the position that the distinction between two these two classes of delusion is real and perhaps even fundamental.

Duality is again evident at the psychological level of analysis, this time as the two factor theory. On the face of it, this duality seems completely different from the above phenomenological one, having nothing to do with questions of meaning and significance. However, the connection might be closer than it first appears, because, as argued at the end of Chapter 7, Coltheart and co-workers' second factor may be relevant not just to monothematic delusions in neurological disease but might also serve as a basis for understanding the class of propositional delusions that arise in response to other pathological experiences, from depressed mood, to auditory hallucinations, to Frith's (1992) proposed failure to label self-generated movements as one's own. It might even be that the second factor has a broader reach still, saying something about the nature of propositional delusions generally – after all, what is the privileging of certain items of information that arrive in conscious awareness so that they do not need to be subjected to fact-checking, if not a description of what it is to be deluded?

At the level of brain function a candidate for duality also exists, in terms of the two different roles that mesotelencephalic dopamine appears to fulfil. On the one hand, it provides the signal necessary for neutral stimuli that predict reward to acquire motivational and reinforcing properties. On the other, it has some not very well characterized facilitatory influence on voluntary motor behaviour. The former translates, via aberrant salience, into referentiality. Can the latter function somehow be made to serve as a theory of propositional delusions? Disregarding some hand-waving by Gray et al. (1991) about the programming of selective attention, the answer seems to be no – it seems highly improbable that the gulf between motor function and cognition can ever be bridged conceptually. What is possible, however, is that that if dopamine has two different functions, it might also have a third, especially when it is remembered that the mesotelencephalic dopamine system projects not only to parts of the basal ganglia with motor and reward functions, but also to many other brain regions. Some speculation about what form such a further function might take is indulged in later on in this chapter.

Delusions: Strictly Personal?

A feature of delusions that has been given short shrift over the years is the fact that, in the vast majority of cases, they concern the patients themselves or people close to them. Deluded patients may say 'I am Jesus' or 'the Mafia are persecuting me', or occasionally that 'my wife has been replaced by an impostor', but they do not on the whole develop beliefs about their bank manager being Jesus, or the Mafia persecuting a friend of theirs, or the man-down-the-street's wife having been replaced by a double. Impersonal delusions are certainly seen, as in the patients described in Chapter 1 who believed that England's coast was melting or that there was an international conspiracy to get rid of people involving lifts and sausage machines (and perhaps also in Laws et al.'s (1995) patient described in Chapter 5, who believed that the British politician David Steel had stood in Italian elections and that another British politician, David Owen, was the leader of the Scientologists) – but these seem to be the exception rather than the rule. Nor is this point trivial since, as described in Chapter 4, being personal rather than impersonal is a key characteristic that distinguishes delusions from the forms of false belief seen in healthy people.

As noted in Chapter 5, this observation maps neatly onto a well-established division at the psychological level, to the extent that delusions can almost be said to have a particular cognitive address in personal semantic memory (albeit blurring into the remainder of semantic memory and episodic memory in severe illness). Following the Fletcher and Frith scheme, the theme of person-centredness should also be reprised at the neurobiological level. And in a way it is: salience theory, the leading (and currently the only) brain-based theory of delusions, has its roots in animal learning theory. However, everything (or perhaps more accurately almost everything) that animals learn, they learn from their own experience; they have little or nothing in the way of an ability to acquire information in the way humans do, by receiving it directly from others. In a very real sense, then, knowledge in this sense is personal. Or to put it in a way that is also picked up again later in this chapter, it is prelinguistic.

Putting Flesh on the Bones

A summary of the conclusions reached so far might run as follows. The concept of aberrant salience, the inappropriate acquisition of motivational and reinforcing properties by neutral stimuli, provides a powerful and intuitive way of understanding referential delusions. Although the empirical evidence suggests that salience is reduced rather than exaggerated in patients with psychotic symptoms, this is not as damaging as a finding of no change, and so the theory perhaps ought not to be cast into the outer darkness just yet. Out of a number of approaches to propositional delusions, the only one that survives is Coltheart and co-workers' proposal of dysfunction in a system that automatically fact-checks information arriving in conscious awareness. Evidence in support of this theory is almost entirely lacking, and there are questions as to why such a counter-intuitive cognitive process should exist in the first place. Nevertheless, the theory has the virtue of being the product of an extended period of logical deduction, and it also seems almost certain that something similar underlies the related phenomenon of confabulation.

In Chapter 7 it was argued that Coltheart and co-workers' conceptualization of the second factor – as inappropriate labelling of information entering awareness with feeling of rightness – could not be a deficit (although they hedged their bets with the alternative possibility of failure to assign a feeling of doubt). If this argument is correct, then the two components of a minimal model of delusions start to inch towards to each other: referential delusions are the result of aberrant salience and propositional delusions of what might be termed aberrant feeling of rightness.

Needless to say, formidable problems remain. Not least among these is that the interaction between aberrant salience and aberrant feeling of rightness needs to be such that it does not lead to a prediction that referential delusions are a precondition for propositional delusions. At the same time, however, the two processes cannot be completely divorced from each other. If this were so, it would mean that delusions are the result of two different pathological processes that just happen to be going on at the same time. Logic, not to mention Occam's razor, demands that both aberrant salience and aberrant feeling of rightness (if this is what turns out to underlie propositional delusions) should be the manifestations of what is at some deeper level the same abnormality.

If, as it probably is, aberrant salience is the result of a dopamine excess, could it be that the same neurochemical abnormality is responsible for aberrant feeling of rightness? Given, as mentioned earlier, that the mesotelencephalic dopamine system extends to brain regions far beyond the dorsal and ventral striatum, this is a not unreasonable position to take. There seems no reason why, say, the arrival of a reward prediction error signal in the ventral striatum might not simultaneously be accompanied by a message marking this occurrence in other parts of the brain, perhaps those concerned with building predictive models of the world. Further speculation on what the nature of this message might be entails going back to Gray's (1981) theory of septo-hippocampal function (minus the part about the hippocampus). In his theory the modulatory transmitters noradrenalin and serotonin were involved in the registration of novelty, punishment and non-reward, and served to label stimuli as 'important, check carefully'. Could it be that dopamine acts to label stimuli associated with reward in some kind of inverse way, perhaps as 'no need to stop and consider', or possibly even as 'privileged'?

Of course, this whole line of reasoning depends on the dopamine hypothesis of schizophrenia being correct, and it may still be wrong, or possibly continue in the kind of limbo that has characterized its history so far. Even if it does turn out to be wrong, all is not lost. The studies described in Chapter 6 make it clear that inducing delusions in normal volunteers is not the exclusive preserve of dopamine agonist drugs, and referentiality in particular can be produced by a variety of other pharmacological interventions. Perhaps the time has come to start to broaden the argument from salience to the brain mechanisms of learning and memory, as achieved by means of synaptic plasticity.

Last but not Least: How Referential and Propositional Delusions Might Be Related

At the phenomenological level, the relationship between referential and propositional delusions is one of partial dissociation. Clinical observations going back to the time of Kraepelin and Bleuler make it clear that while propositional delusions often develop as an explanation of earlier referential delusions, this is not always the case, either in schizophrenia or in delusional disorder, and perhaps even less so in psychotic forms of depression and mania. Is there anything more that can be said about this relationship, perhaps within Fletcher and Frith's (2009) framework?

The thoughts of two groups of authors may be relevant here. The first is Corlett et al. (2010b) theorizing about the requirements for predictive models of the world in the context of learning theory:

> [T]o navigate the world successfully, we must sustain a set of prior beliefs (our internal model), sufficiently robust that we do not react reflexively and chaotically to any incoming sensory stimulus. At the same time, these beliefs (priors) must not be so immutable that our responses become fixed, stereotypical and insensitive to change.

Arguing at a completely different level, as part of their attempt to account for the Capgras delusion, Stone and Young (1997) brought up a philosophical distinction between two processes that appear to operate in the formation and revision of beliefs. On the one hand, there is the principle of conservatism, which refers to the normal tendency to try and explain new events in terms of existing knowledge and avoid introducing new concepts willy nilly. This tendency is in constant tension with another principle, observational adequacy, the need to do justice to novel and unexpected events that challenge existing beliefs. The way in which one or other of these two opposing tendencies gain the upper hand was illustrated by Davies and Coltheart (2000) using two hypothetical scenarios involving unexpected events. The first concerned one of the authors seeing a mouse in the corner of his office, located in the Coombs Building. While this observation might be in conflict with prior assumptions about the level of pest control to be expected in universities, the right course of action is clearly to accept the experience and update his previous beliefs on the matter accordingly. Davies and Coltheart (2000) then went on to outline another scenario:

> But suppose that, sitting in my office, I seem to see in the corner several little green men playing blackjack with a pink elephant dealing the cards. It might be that I antecedently have an explicitly articulated and compelling set of reasons for believing that there are no blackjack-dealing pink elephants in the Coombs Building. Or it might be that, although I have never set out to construct an explicit justification, the proposition that my office is not populated by green men and pink elephants figures as an implicit background assumption in my assessments of the way in which evidence confirms or disconfirms hypotheses. Either way, if I accept my experience as veridical and try to incorporate the 'little green men and a pink elephant' hypothesis into my system of beliefs then very substantial disruption will result. Here, the principle of conservatism outweighs the principle of observational adequacy and dictates that I should not take my experience at face value. I should deny the apparent data.

At first sight, what both Corlett et al. (2010b) and Stone and Young (1997)/Davies and Coltheart (2000) are saying seems to be similar: a dynamic interaction has to exist between models of the world and events that do not conform to them. However, there is also a difference, in that while for Corlett and co-workers the process of forming predictions and updating them are two sides of the same coin – predictions about events are built up from what is experienced and constantly compared with this, with errors being used to modify the original prediction – there is no such requirement in the case of conservatism and observational adequacy. They could be entirely independent cognitive processes with different sources of input, and perhaps carried out at different levels of brain organization.

It might not be going too far to suppose that if these two processes were different, the distinction between them might involve language. Animals form and modify predictions using processes which are by definition non-linguistic and which, according to Friston (2010), may represent a general mode of central nervous system functioning. Humans, however, also possess a parallel system for updating their predictions about the world, which is language-based and so will inevitably operate according to different rules. When the first system malfunctions, the result would be an essentially prelinguistic experience, delusional mood (or as this book would argue, referentiality more generally). When the second system malfunctions, perhaps on the basis of receiving incorrect and uncorrectable information from the first system (but also, it would have to be proposed, on the basis of some as yet unknown disturbance as well), the result might be propositional delusions. To put it another way, referential delusions are the result of abnormality in the world as it is experienced whereas propositional delusions involve the world as it is known.

This is the argument recently made by Hinzen et al. (2016) in a theoretical exploration of the possibility that delusions are a linguistic phenomenon. While what the authors propose might be considered to be at the outer limits of reasonable speculation, such an argument does have one undeniable advantage – invoking language brings with it the possibility of senses of meaning beyond simply that of stimuli having significance for behaviour. One well-known form of meaning that exists at the linguistic level is semantics, the meaning of words. This does not seem particularly relevant to delusions – as Hinzen et al. (2016) point out, when deluded patients say they are Jesus, or that the Mafia are persecuting them, they are using words in the same way as everyone else and we know exactly what they mean. However, there is also another type of linguistic meaning, which is well recognized, particularly in philosophy, that of propositional meaning. This is the kind of meaning that arises from grammatical structuring of lexical-semantic information when the level of complexity of full sentences is reached. Furthermore, it is generally accepted in philosophical circles that it is this form of meaning which gives statements their quality of being true or false. With this, a point might finally have been reached where Jaspers' (1959) proposal that all kinds of delusions, not just referential delusions, represent a change in meaning might not seem so strange after all.

References

Aaronovitch, D. (2010). *Voodoo Histories: How Conspiracy Theory Has Shaped Modern History*. London: Vintage.

Abi-Dargham, A., Gil, R., Krystal, J. et al. (1998). Increased striatal dopamine transmission in schizophrenia: confirmation in a second cohort. *American Journal of Psychiatry*, 155, 761–767.

Abraham, W. C., & Williams, J. M. (2003). Properties and mechanisms of LTP maintenance. *The Neuroscientist*, 9, 463–474.

Adams, R. A., Stephan, K. E., Brown, H. R., Frith, C. D., & Friston, K. J. (2013). The computational anatomy of psychosis. *Frontiers in Psychiatry*, 4, 47.

Adler, C. M., Goldberg, T. E., Malhotra, A. K., Pickar, D., & Breier, A. (1998). Effects of ketamine on thought disorder, working memory, and semantic memory in healthy volunteers. *Biological Psychiatry*, 43, 811–816.

Adler, C. M., Malhotra, A. K., Elman, I., et al. (1999). Comparison of ketamine-induced thought disorder in healthy volunteers and thought disorder in schizophrenia. *American Journal of Psychiatry*, 156, 1646–1649.

Agnati, L. F., Fuxe, K., Zoli, M. et al. (1986). A correlation analysis of the regional distribution of central enkephalin and beta-endorphin immunoreactive terminals and of opiate receptors in adult and old male rats. Evidence for the existence of two main types of communication in the central nervous system: the volume transmission and the wiring transmission. *Acta Physiologica Scandinavica*, 128, 201–207.

Agnati, L. F., Zoli, M., Stromberg, I., & Fuxe, K. (1995). Intercellular communication in the brain: wiring versus volume transmission. *Neuroscience*, 69, 711–726.

Agnati, L. F., Guidolin, D., Guescini, M., Genedani, S., & Fuxe, K. (2010). Understanding wiring and volume transmission. *Brain Research Reviews*, 64, 137–159.

Alexander, G. E., DeLong, M. R., & Strick, P. L. (1986). Parallel organization of functionally segregated circuits linking basal ganglia and cortex. *Annual Review of Neuroscience*, 9, 357–381.

Alexander, M. P., Stuss, D. T., & Benson, D. F. (1979). Capgras syndrome: a reduplicative phenomenon. *Neurology*, 29, 334–339.

Andreasen, N. C. (1982). Negative symptoms in schizophrenia. Definition and reliability. *Archives of General Psychiatry*, 39, 784–788.

Andreasen, N. C., & Bardach, J. (1977). Dysmorphophobia: symptom or disease? *American Journal of Psychiatry*, 134, 673–676.

Andreasen, N. C., & Olsen, S. (1982). Negative v positive schizophrenia. Definition and validation. *Archives of General Psychiatry*, 39, 789–794.

Andreasen, N. C., Arndt, S., Alliger, R., Miller, D., & Flaum, M. (1995). Symptoms of schizophrenia. Methods, meanings, and mechanisms. *Archives of General Psychiatry*, 52, 341–351.

Angrist, B. M., & Gershon, S. (1970). The phenomenology of experimentally induced amphetamine psychosis – preliminary observations. *Biological Psychiatry*, 2, 95–107.

Angrist, B., & Sudilovsky, A. (1978). Central nervous system stimulants: historical aspects and clinical effects. In L. L. Iversen, S. E. Iversen & S. H. Snyder (Eds.), *Handbook of Psychopharmacology, Volume 11, Stimulants* (pp. 99–166). New York: Plenum.

Arseneault, L., Cannon, M., Witton, J., & Murray, R. M. (2004). Causal association between cannabis and psychosis: examination of the evidence. *British Journal of Psychiatry*, 184, 110–117.

Aziz, V. M., & Warner, N. J. (2005). Capgras' syndrome of time. *Psychopathology*, 38, 49–52.

Babinski, J. (1914). Contribution à l'étude des troubles mentaux dans l'hémiplégie organique-cérébrale (Anosognosie). *Revue Neurologique*, 27, 845–847.

Babinski, J. (1918). Anosognosie. *Revue Neurologique (Paris)*. 31, 365–367.

Baddeley, A., & Wilson, B. (1988). Frontal amnesia and the dysexecutive syndrome. *Brain and Cognition*, 7, 212–230.

Badie, D. (2010). Groupthink, Iraq, and the war on terror: explaining US policy shift toward Iraq. *Foreign Policy Analysis*, 6, 277–296.

Barkun, M. (2013). *A Culture of Conspiracy: Apocalyptic Visions in Contemporary America, 2nd Edition*. Berkeley and Los Angeles: University of California Press.

Baruk, H. (1959). Delusions of passion. Translated (1974). In S. R. Hirsch & M. Shepherd (Eds.), *Themes and Variations in European Psychiatry* (pp. 375–384). Bristol: Wright.

Basso, M. R., Nasrallah, H. A., Olson, S. C., & Bornstein, R. A. (1998). Neuropsychological correlates of negative, disorganized and psychotic symptoms in schizophrenia. *Schizophrenia Research*, 31, 99–111.

Bauer, R. M. (1984). Autonomic recognition of names and faces in prosopagnosia: a neuropsychological application of the Guilty Knowledge Test. *Neuropsychologia*, 22, 457–469.

Baxter, R. D., & Liddle, P. F. (1998). Neuropsychological deficits associated with schizophrenic syndromes. *Schizophrenia Research*, 30, 239–249.

Bayne, T., & Pacherie, E. (2005). In defence of the doxastic conception of delusions. *Mind and Language*, 20, 163–188.

Bear, M. F., & Malenka, R. C. (1994). Synaptic plasticity: LTP and LTD. *Current Opinion in Neurobiology*, 4, 389–399.

Beck, A. T. (1967). *Depression: Causes and Treatment*. Philadelphia: University of Pennsylvania Press.

Beck, A. T. (1979). Meaning and emotions. In A. T. Beck (Ed.), *Cognitive Therapy and the Emotional Disorders* (pp. 47–75). London: Penguin.

Beck, A. T. (2008). The evolution of the cognitive model of depression and its neurobiological correlates. *American Journal of Psychiatry*, 165, 969–977.

Begum, M., & McKenna, P. J. (2011). Olfactory reference syndrome: a systematic review of the world literature. *Psychological Medicine*, 41, 453–461.

Bell, M. D., Lysaker, P. H., Milstein, R. M., & Beam-Goulet, J. L. (1994). Concurrent validity of the cognitive component of schizophrenia: relationship of PANSS scores to neuropsychological assessments. *Psychiatry Research*, 54, 51–58.

Beninger, R. J. (1983). The role of dopamine in locomotor activity and learning. *Brain Research*, 287, 173–196.

Benson, D. F., Gardner, H., & Meadows, J. C. (1976). Reduplicative paramnesia. *Neurology*, 26, 147–151.

Berridge, K. C. (2007). The debate over dopamine's role in reward: the case for incentive salience. *Psychopharmacology*, 191, 391–431.

Berridge, K. C., & Robinson, T. E. (1998). What is the role of dopamine in reward: hedonic impact, reward learning, or incentive salience? *Brain Research: Brain Research Reviews*, 28, 309–369.

Berrios, G. E. (1998). Confabulations: a conceptual history. *Journal of the History of Neuroscience*, 7, 225–241.

Bhatia, M. S. (1990). Capgras syndrome in a patient with migraine. *British Journal of Psychiatry*, 157, 917–918.

Bisiach, E., & Geminiani, G. (1991). Anosognosia related to hemiplegia and hemianopia. In G. P. Prigatano & D. L. Schacter (Eds.), *Awareness of Deficit after Brain Injury* (pp. 17–39). New York/Oxford: Oxford University Press.

Bjork, J. M., Knutson, B., Fong, G. W. et al. (2004). Incentive-elicited brain activation in adolescents: similarities and differences from young adults. *Journal of Neuroscience*, 24, 1793–1802.

Bjorklund, A., & Dunnett, S. B. (2007). Dopamine neuron systems in the brain: an update. *Trends in Neurosciences*, 30, 194–202.

Bjorklund, A., & Lindvall, O. (1984). Dopamine-containing systems in the CNS. In A. Bjorklund & T. Hokfelt (Eds.), *Handbook of Chemical Neuroanatomy, Volume 2*. Amsterdam: Elsevier.

Blakemore, S. J., Sarfati, Y., Bazin, N., & Decety, J. (2003). The detection of intentional contingencies in simple animations in patients with delusions of persecution. *Psychological Medicine*, 33, 1433–1441.

Blashfield, R. K. (1984). *The Classification of Psychopathology: Neo-Kraepelian and Quantitative Approaches*. New York: Plenum.

Bleuler, E. (1911). *Dementia Praecox or the Group of Schizophrenias* (translated by J. Zinkin, 1950). New York: International Universities Press.

Bleuler, E. (1924). *Textbook of Psychiatry* (translated by A. A. Brill, 1951). London: George Allen and Unwin.

Bliss, T. V., & Collingridge, G. L. (1993). A synaptic model of memory: long-term potentiation in the hippocampus. *Nature*, 361, 31–39.

Blom, R. M., Hennekam, R. C., & Denys, D. (2012). Body integrity identity disorder. *PLoS One*, 7, e34702.

Bloom, F. E. (1984). General features of chemically identified neurons. In A. Bjorklund & T. Hokfelt (Eds.), *Handbook of Chemical Neuroanatomy, Volume 2*. Amsterdam: Elsevier.

Bora, E., Yucel, M., & Pantelis, C. (2009). Theory of mind impairment in schizophrenia: meta-analysis. *Schizophrenia Research*, 109, 1–9.

Bosch, M., & Hayashi, Y. (2012). Structural plasticity of dendritic spines. *Current Opinion in Neurobiology*, 22, 383–388.

Bowdle, T. A., Radant, A. D., Cowley, D. S. et al. (1998). Psychedelic effects of ketamine in healthy volunteers: relationship to steady-state plasma concentrations. *Anesthesiology*, 88, 82–88.

Bowers, M. B., Jr. (1968). Pathogenesis of acute schizophrenic psychosis. An experimental approach. *Archives of General Psychiatry*, 19, 348–355.

Bowers, M. B., Jr., & Freedman, D. X. (1966). 'Psychedelic' experiences in acute psychoses. *Archives of General Psychiatry*, 15, 240–248.

Box, O., Laing, H., & Kopelman, M. (1999). The evolution of spontaneous confabulation, delusional misidentification and a related delusion in a case of severe head injury. *Neurocase*, 5, 251–262.

Breier, A., Su, T. P., Saunders, R. et al. (1997). Schizophrenia is associated with elevated amphetamine-induced synaptic dopamine concentrations: evidence from a novel positron emission tomography method. *Proceedings of the National Academy of Sciences U S A*, 94, 2569–2574.

Brekke, J. S., DeBonis, J. A., & Graham, J. W. (1994). A latent structure analysis of the positive and negative symptoms in schizophrenia. *Comprehensive Psychiatry*, 35, 252–259.

Brekke, J. S., Raine, A., & Thomson, C. (1995). Cognitive and psychophysiological correlates of positive, negative, and disorganized symptoms in the schizophrenia spectrum. *Psychiatry Research*, 57, 241–250.

Brotherton, R. A. (2013). *Measurement Issues and the Role of Cognitive Biases in Conspiracist Ideation*. (PhD), Unpublished PhD thesis, University of London.

Brotherton, R. (2015). *Suspicious Minds: Why We Believe Conspiracy Theories*. New York/London: Bloomsbury Sigma.

Brown, K. W., & White, T. (1992). Syndromes of chronic schizophrenia and some clinical correlates. *British Journal of Psychiatry*, 161, 317–322.

Brüne, M., & Brüne-Cohrs, U. (2006). Theory of mind–evolution, ontogeny, brain mechanisms and psychopathology. *Neuroscience and Biobehavoral Reviews*, 30, 437–455.

Buchanan, R. W., Javitt, D. C., Marder, S. R. et al. (2007). The cognitive and negative symptoms in schizophrenia trial (CONSIST): the efficacy of glutamatergic agents for negative symptoms and cognitive impairments. *American Journal of Psychiatry*, 164, 1593–1602.

Buck, K. D., Waramn, D. M., Huddy, V., & Lysaker, P. H. (2012). The relationship of metacognition with jumping to conclusions among persons with schizophrenia spectrum disorders. *Psychopathology*, 45, 271–275.

Burgess, P. W., & McNeil, J. E. (1999). Content-specific confabulation. *Cortex*, 35, 163–182.

Burgess, P. W., & Shallice, T. (1996). Confabulation and the control of recollection. *Memory*, 4, 359–411.

Burgess, P. W., Baxter, D., Rose, M., & Alderman, N. (1996). Delusional paramnesic misidentification. In P. W. Halligan & J. C. Marshall (Eds.), *Methods in Madness* (pp. 51–78). Hove: Psychology Press.

Burgy, M. (2007). Obsession in the strict sense: a helpful psychopathological phenomenon in the differential diagnosis between obsessive-compulsive disorder and schizophrenia. *Psychopathology*, 40, 102–110.

Bush, R. R., & Mosteller, F. (1951a). A mathematical model for simple learning. *Psychological Review*, 58, 313–323.

Bush, R. R., & Mosteller, F. (1951b). A model for stimulus generalization and discrimination. *Psychological Review*, 58, 413–423.

Cadenhead, K. (2014). Worried and oddly preoccupied. In J. W. Barnhill (Ed.), *DSM-5™ Clinical Cases* (pp. 306–308). Washington, DC: American Psychiatric Publishing.

Cadenhead, K. S., Geyer, M. A., Butler, R. W. et al. (1997). Information processing deficits of schizophrenia patients: relationship to clinical ratings, gender and medication status. *Schizophrenia Research*, 28, 51–62.

Cameron, A. M., Oram, J., Geffen, G. M. et al. (2002). Working memory correlates of three symptom clusters in schizophrenia. *Psychiatry Research*, 110, 49–61.

Cashman, F. E., & Pollock, B. (1983). Treatment of monosymptomatic hypochondriacal psychosis with imipramine. *Canadian Journal of Psychiatry*, 28, 85.

Catapano, F., Sperandeo, R., Perris, F., Lanzaro, M., & Maj, M. (2001). Insight and resistance in patients with obsessive-compulsive disorder. *Psychopathology*, 34, 62–68.

Catts, V. S., Lai, Y. L., Weickert, C. S., Weickert, T. W., & Catts, S. V. (2016). A quantitative review of the postmortem evidence for decreased cortical n-methyl-d-aspartate receptor expression levels in schizophrenia: how can we link molecular abnormalities to mismatch negativity deficits? *Biological Psychology*, 116, 57–67.

Chapanis, N. P., & Chapanis, A. (1964). Cognitive dissonance: five years later. *Psychological Bulletin*, 61, 1–22.

Chen, C. K., Lin, S. K., Sham, P. C. et al. (2003). Pre-morbid characteristics and co-morbidity of methamphetamine users with and without psychosis. *Psychological Medicine*, 33, 1407–1414.

Chen, E. Y., Wilkins, A. J., & McKenna, P. J. (1994). Semantic memory is both impaired and anomalous in schizophrenia. *Psychological Medicine*, 24, 193–202.

Citri, A., & Malenka, R. C. (2008). Synaptic plasticity: multiple forms, functions, and mechanisms. *Neuropsychopharmacology*, 33, 18–41.

Clancy, M. J., Clarke, M. C., Connor, D. J., Cannon, M., & Cotter, D. R. (2014). The prevalence of psychosis in epilepsy; a systematic review and meta-analysis. *BMC Psychiatry*, 14, 75.

Clark, O., & O'Carroll, R. E. (1998). An examination of the relationship between executive function, memory and rehabilitation status in schizophrenia. *Neuropsychological Rehabilitation*, 8, 229–241.

Clérambault, G. G. (1942). *Oeuvres Psychiatriques*. Paris: P.U.F.

Cobb, J. (1979). Morbid jealousy. *British Journal of Hospital Medicine*, 21, 511–518.

Cocchini, G., Beschin, N., & Sala, S. D. (2002). Chronic anosognosia: a case report and theoretical account. *Neuropsychologia*, 40, 2030–2038.

Colbert, S. M., Peters, E., & Garety, P. (2010). Jumping to conclusions and perceptions in early psychosis: relationship with delusional beliefs. *Cognitive Neuropsychiatry*, 15, 422–440.

Collins, A. M. & Quillian, M. R. (1969). Retrieval time from semantic memory. *Journal of Verbal Learning and Verbal Behavior*, 8, 240–247.

Coltheart, M. (2005). Conscious experience and delusional belief. *Philosophy, Psychiatry and Psychology*, 12, 153–157.

Coltheart, M., Langdon, R., & McKay, R. (2007). Schizophrenia and monothematic delusions. *Schizophrenia Bulletin*, 33, 642–647.

Coltheart, M., Langdon, R., & McKay, R. (2011). Delusional belief. *Annual Review of Psychology*, 62, 271–298.

Connell, P. (1958). *Amphetamine Psychosis, Maudsley Monograph, No. 5*. London: Oxford University Press.

Corcoran, R., & Frith, C. D. (1996). Conversational conduct and the symptoms of schizophrenia. *Cognitive Neuropsychiatry*, 1, 305–318.

Corcoran, R., Cahill, C., & Frith C. D. (1997). The appreciation of visual jokes in people with schizophrenia: a study of 'mentalizing' ability. *Schizophrenia Research*, 11, 319–327.

Corcoran, R., Mercer, G., & Frith, C. D. (1995). Schizophrenia, symptomatology and social inference: investigating "theory of mind" in people with schizophrenia. *Schizophr Research*, 17, 5–13.

Corlett, P. R., D'Souza, D. C., & Krystal, J. H. (2010a). Capgras syndrome induced by ketamine in a healthy subject. *Biological Psychiatry*, 68, e1–2.

Corlett, P. R., Frith, C. D., & Fletcher, P. C. (2009). From drugs to deprivation: a Bayesian framework for understanding models of psychosis. *Psychopharmacology (Berlin)*, 206, 515–530.

Corlett, P. R., Taylor, J. R., Wang, X. J., Fletcher, P. C., & Krystal, J. H. (2010b). Toward a neurobiology of delusions. *Progress in Neurobiology*, 92, 345–369.

Coyle, F. A., Jr., & Bernard, J. L. (1965). Logical thinking and paranoid schizophrenia. *Journal of Psychology*, 60, 283–289.

Coyne, J. C. (1989). Thinking postcognitively about depression. In A. Freeman, K. Simon, L. Beutler & H. Arkowitz (Eds.), *Comprehensive Handbook of Cognitive Therapy* (pp. 227–244). New York: Plenum.

Critchley, M. (1953). *The Parietal Lobes*. London: Arnold.

Crow, T. J. (1980). Molecular pathology of schizophrenia: more than one disease process? *British Medical Journal*, 280, 66–68.

Cuesta, M. J., & Peralta, V. (1995). Cognitive disorders in the positive, negative, and disorganization syndromes of schizophrenia. *Psychiatry Research*, 58, 227–235.

Cummings, J. L. (1991). Behavioral complications of drug treatment of Parkinson's disease. *Journal of the American Geriatrics Society*, 39, 708–716.

Cutting, J. (1978). Study of anosognosia. *Journal of Neurology, Neurosurgery and Psychiatry*, 41, 548–555.

Cutting, J. (1980). Physical illness and psychosis. *British Journal of Psychiatry*, 136, 109–119.

Cutting, J. (1985). *The Psychology of Schizophrenia*. Edinburgh: Churchill Livingstone.

Daban, C., Amado, I., Bayle, F. et al. (2002). Correlation between clinical syndromes and neuropsychological tasks in unmedicated patients with recent onset schizophrenia. *Psychiatry Research*, 113, 83–92.

Damasio, A. R., Graff-Radford, N. R., Eslinger, P. J., Damasio, H., & Kassell, N. (1985). Amnesia following basal forebrain lesions. *Archives of Neurology*, 42, 263–271.

David, A. S. (1999). On the impossibility of defining delusions. *Philosophy, Psychiatry, and Psychology*, 6, 17–20.

David, A. S. (2010). Why we need more debate on whether psychotic symptoms lie on a continuum with normality. *Psychological Medicine*, 40, 1935–1942.

David, A. S., & Prince, M. (2005). Psychosis following head injury: a critical review. *Journal of Neurology, Neurosurgery and Psychiatry*, 76 Suppl 1, i53–60.

Davies, B. M., & Beech, H. R. (1960). The effect of 1-arylcylohexylamine (sernyl) on twelve normal volunteers. *Journal of Mental Science*, 106, 912–924.

Davies, M. A., & Coltheart, M. (2000). Introduction: pathologies of belief. *Mind and Language*, 15, 1–46.

Davies, M., Davies, A. M., & Coltheart, M. (2005). Anosognosia and the two-factor theory of delusions. *Mind and Language*, 20, 209–236.

Davison, K., & Bagley, C. R. (1969). Schizophrenia-like psychoses associated with organic disorders of the central nervous system: a review. *British Journal of Psychiatry, Special Publication* 4, 113–183.

de Leon, J., Bott, A., & Simpson, G. M. (1989). Dysmorphophobia: body dysmorphic disorder or delusional disorder, somatic subtype? *Comprehensive Psychiatry*, 30, 457–472.

de Pauw, K. W., Szulecka, T. K., & Poltock, T. L. (1987). Fregoli syndrome after cerebral infarction. *Journal of Nervous and Mental Disease*, 175, 433–438.

de Portugal, E., Martinez, C., Gonzalez, N. et al. (2011). Clinical and cognitive correlates of psychiatric comorbidity in delusional disorder outpatients. *Australia and New Zealand Journal of Psychiatry*, 45, 416–425.

Delespaul, P., & van Os, J. (2003). Jaspers was right after all – delusions are distinct from normal beliefs. Against. *British Journal of Psychiatry*, 183, 286.

DeLuca, J. (1993). Predicting neurobehavioral patterns following anterior communicating artery aneurysm. *Cortex*, 29, 639–647.

Dibben, C. R., Rice, C., Laws, K., & McKenna, P. J. (2009). Is executive impairment associated with schizophrenic syndromes? A meta-analysis. *Psychological Medicine*, 39, 381–392.

Dollfus, S., & Everitt, B. (1998). Symptom structure in schizophrenia: two-, three- or four-factor models? *Psychopathology*, 31, 120–130.

Doody, G. A., Götz, M., Johnstone, E. C., Frith, C.D., & Owens DG. (1998). Theory of mind and psychoses. *Psychological Medicine*, 28, 397–405.

Doughty, O. J., & Done, D. J. (2009). Is semantic memory impaired in schizophrenia? A systematic review and meta-analysis of 91 studies. *Cognitive Neuropsychiatry*, 14, 473–509.

Draycott, S., & Dabbs, A. (1998). Cognitive Dissonance. 1: an overview of the literature and its integration into theory and practice in clinical psychology. *British Journal of Clinical Psychology*, 37, 341–353.

D'Souza, D. C., Perry, E., MacDougall, L. et al. (2004). The psychotomimetic effects of intravenous delta-9-tetrahydrocannabinol

in healthy individuals: implications for psychosis. *Neuropsychopharmacology*, 29, 1558–1572.

Dudley, R., Shaftoe, D., Cavanagh, K. et al. (2011). 'Jumping to conclusions' in first-episode psychosis. *Early Intervention Psychiatry*, 5, 50–56.

Dudley, R., Taylor, P., Wickham, S., & Hutton, P. (2016). Psychosis, delusions and the 'jumping to conclusions' reasoning bias: a systematic review and meta-analysis. *Schizophrenia Bulletin*, 42, 652–665.

Earleywine, M. (2002). *Understanding Marijuana*. Oxford: Oxford University Press.

Eberle, P. (2003). *The Abuse of Innocence: The McMartin Preschool Trial*. Amherst, NY: Prometheus Books.

Eckman, P. S., & Shean, G. D. (2000). Impairment in test performance and symptom dimensions of schizophrenia. *Journal of Psychiatric Research*, 34, 147–153.

Edelstyn, N. M., & Oyebode, F. (1999). A review of the phenomenology and cognitive neuropsychological origins of the Capgras syndrome. *International Journal of Geriatric Psychiatry*, 14, 48–59.

Egerton, A., Chaddock, C. A., Winton-Brown, T. T. et al. (2013). Presynaptic striatal dopamine dysfunction in people at ultra-high risk for psychosis: findings in a second cohort. *Biological Psychiatry*, 74, 106–112.

Eisen, J. L., & Rasmussen, S. A. (1993). Obsessive compulsive disorder with psychotic features. *Journal of Clinical Psychiatry*, 54, 373–379.

Ellis, H. D., & Young, A. W. (1990). Accounting for delusional misidentifications. *British Journal of Psychiatry*, 157, 239–248.

Ellis, H. D., Whitley, J., & Luaute, J. P. (1994). Delusional misidentification. The three original papers on the Capgras, Fregoli and intermetamorphosis delusions. (Classic Text No. 17). *History of Psychiatry*, 5, 117–146.

Ellis, H. D., Young, A. W., Quayle, A. H., & De Pauw, K. W. (1997). Reduced autonomic responses to faces in Capgras delusion. *Proceedings of the Royal Society B: Biological Sciences*, 264, 1085–1092.

Enoch, M. D., & Ball, H. N. (2001). *Uncommon Psychiatric Syndromes, 4th Edition.* London/ New York/New Delhi: Arnold.

Enoch, M. D., Trethowan, W. H., & Barker, J. C. (1967). *Some Uncommon Psychiatric Syndromes.* Bristol: Wright.

Falcone, M. A., Murray, R. M., Wiffen, B. D. et al. (2015). Jumping to conclusions, neuropsychological functioning, and delusional beliefs in first episode psychosis. *Schizophrenia Bulletin*, 41, 411–418.

Farde, L., Wiesel, F. A., Stone-Elander, S. et al. (1990). D2 dopamine receptors in neuroleptic-naive schizophrenic patients. A positron emission tomography study with [11C]raclopride. *Archives of General Psychiatry*, 47, 213–219.

Feinberg, T. E., Eaton, L.A., Roane, D. M., & Giacino, J. T. (1999). Multiple Fregoli delusions after traumatic brain injury. *Cortex*, 35, 373–387.

Festinger, L., Riecken, H. W., & Schachter, S. (1956). *When Prophecy Fails: A Social and Psychological Study of a Modern Group That Predicted the Destruction of the World.* Minneapolis, MN: University of Minnesota Press.

First, M. B. (2005). Desire for amputation of a limb: paraphilia, psychosis, or a new type of identity disorder. *Psychological Medicine*, 35, 919–928.

First, M. B., & Fisher, C. E. (2012). Body integrity identity disorder: the persistent desire to acquire a physical disability. *Psychopathology*, 45, 3–14.

First, M. B., Spitzer, R. L., Gibbon, M., & Williams, J. B. W. (2002). *The Structured Clinical Interview for DSM-IV Axis I Disorders (Research Version).* New York: Biometrics Research, New York State Psychiatric Institute.

Fischer, R. S., Alexander, M. P., D'Esposito, M., & Otto, R. (1995). Neuropsychological and neuroanatomical correlates of confabulation. *Journal of Clinical and Experimental Neuropsychology*, 17, 20–28.

Fischhoff, B., & Beyth-Marom, R. (1983). Hypothesis evaluation from a Bayesian perspective. *Psychological Review*, 90 239–260.

Fletcher, P. C., & Frith, C. D. (2009). Perceiving is believing: a Bayesian approach to explaining the positive symptoms of schizophrenia. *Nature Reviews Neuroscience*, 10, 48–58.

Foa, E. B. (1979). Failure in treating obsessive-compulsives. *Behaviour Research and Therapy*, 17, 169–176.

Foa, E. B., Kozak, M. J., Goodman, W. K. et al. (1995). DSM-IV field trial: obsessive-compulsive disorder. *American Journal of Psychiatry*, 152, 90–96.

Forrest, A. D. (1975). Paranoid states and paranoid psychoses. In A. Forrest & J. Affleck (Eds.), *New Perspectives in Schizophrenia* (pp. 32–44). Edinburgh: Churchill Livingstone.

Forrest, A.D (1978). Schizophrenia, schizophreniform and paranoid psychosis. In A. D. Forrest, J. W. Affleck & A. K. Zealley (Eds.), *Companion to Psychiatric Studies, 2nd Edition* (pp. 438–458). Edinburgh: Churchill Livingstone.

Förstl, H., Besthorn, C., Burns, A. et al. (1994). Delusional misidentification in Alzheimer's disease: a summary of clinical and biological aspects. *Psychopathology*, 27, 194–199.

Freeman, D. (2007). Suspicious minds: the psychology of persecutory delusions. *Clinical Psychological Review*, 27, 425–457.

Freeman, D., Garety, P. A., Kuipers, E., Fowler, D., & Bebbington, P. E. (2002). A cognitive model of persecutory delusions. *British Journal of Clinical Psychology*, 41, 331–347.

Freeman, D., Startup, H., Dunn, G. et al. (2014). Understanding jumping to conclusions in patients with persecutory delusions: working memory and intolerance of uncertainty. *Psychological Medicine*, 44, 3017–3024.

Friston, K. (2010). The free-energy principle: a unified brain theory? *Nature Reviews Neuroscience*, 11, 127–138.

Frith, C. D. (1992). *The Cognitive Neuropsychology of Schizophrenia.* Hove: Psychology Press.

Frith, C. D. (2004). Schizophrenia and theory of mind. *Psychological Medicine*, 34, 385–389.

Frith, C. D., & Corcoran, R. (1996). Exploring 'theory of mind' in people with schizophrenia. *Psychological Medicine*, 26, 521–530.

Frith, C. D., Blakemore, S. J., & Wolpert, D. M. (2000). Abnormalities in the awareness and control of action. *Philosophical Transactions of the Royal Society B: Biological Sciences*, 355, 1771–1788.

Frith, C. D., Leary, J., Cahill, C., & Johnstone, E. C. (1991). Performance on psychological tests. Demographic and clinical correlates of the results of these tests. *British Journal of Psychiatry*, 159 Supplement 13, 26–29.

Fuxe, K., Dahlstrom, A. B., Jonsson, G., Marcellino, D., Guescini, M., Dam, M., Manger, P., & Agnati, L. (2010). The discovery of central monoamine neurons gave volume transmission to the wired brain. *Progress in Neurobiology*, 90, 82–100.

Garety, P. A., & Freeman, D. (1999). Cognitive approaches to delusions: a critical review of theories and evidence. *British Journal of Clinical Psychology*, 38, 113–154.

Garety, P. A., & Freeman, D. (2013). The past and future of delusions research: from the inexplicable to the treatable. *British Journal of Psychiatry*, 203, 327–333.

Garety, P. A., Kuipers, E., Fowler, D., Freeman, D., & Bebbington, P. E. (2001). A cognitive model of the positive symptoms of psychosis. *Psychological Medicine*, 31, 189–195.

Garety, P., Joyce, E., Jolley, S. et al. (2013). Neuropsychological functioning and jumping to conclusions in delusions. *Schizophrenia Research*, 150, 570–574.

Gilboa, A., & Moscovitch, M. (2002). The cognitive neuroscience of confabulation: a review and model. In A. D. Baddeley, M. D. Kopelman & B. A. Wilson (Eds.), *Handbook of Memory Disorders, 2nd edition* (pp. 315–342). Chichester: Wiley.

Gilboa, A., & Verfaellie, M. (2010). Telling it like it isn't: the cognitive neuroscience of confabulation. *Journal of the Interantional Neuropsychological Society*, 16, 961–966.

Gilboa, A., Alain, C., Stuss, D. T. et al. (2006). Mechanisms of spontaneous confabulations: a strategic retrieval account. *Brain*, 129, 1399–1414.

Gittleson, N. L. (1966). Depressive psychosis in the obsessional neurotic. *British Journal of Psychiatry*, 112, 883–887.

Glimcher, P. W. (2011). Understanding dopamine and reinforcement learning: the dopamine reward prediction error hypothesis. *Proceedings of the National Academy of Sciences USA*, 108 Suppl 3, 15647–15654.

Gluckman, I. K. (1968). A case of Capgras syndrome. *Australian and New Zealand Journal of Psychiatry*, 2, 39–43.

Goertzel, T. (1994). Belief in conspiracy theories. *Political Psychology*, 15, 731–742

Goldberg, G. J. (1965). Obsessional paranoid syndromes. *Psychiatric Quarterly*, 39 43–64.

Gordon, G. (1926). Obsessions in their relation to psychoses. *American Journal of Psychiatry*, 82, 647–659.

Gottesman, L., & Chapman, L. J. (1960). Syllogistic reasoning errors in schizophrenia. *Journal of Consulting Psychology*, 24, 250–255.

Gray, J. A. (1981). *The Neuropsychology of Anxiety: An Enquiry into the Functions of the Septo-Hippocampal System*. Oxford: Clarendon/Oxford University Press.

Gray, J. A. (1998). Integrating schizophrenia. *Schizophrenia Bulletin*, 24, 249–266.

Gray, J. A. (2004). On biology, phenomenology, and pharmacology in schizophrenia. *American Journal of Psychiatry*, 161, 377.

Gray, J. A., Feldon, J., Rawlins, J. N. P., Hemsley, D. R., & Smith, A. D. (1991). The neuropsychology of schizophrenia. *Behavioral and Brain Sciences*, 14, 1–84.

Graybiel, A. M. (2005). The basal ganglia: learning new tricks and loving it. *Current Opinion in Neurobiology*, 15, 638–644.

Griffith, J. D., Cavanaugh, J., & Oates, J. (1968). Paranoid episodes induced by drug. *Journal of the American Medical Association*, 205, 39, 46.

Gross, H., & Kaltenback, E. (1955). Die Anosognosie. *Wiener Zeitschrift für Nervenheilkunde*, 11, 374–418.

Grover, S., Biswas, P., & Avasthi, A. (2007). Delusional disorder: study from North India. *Psychiatry and Clinical Neuroscience*, 61, 462–470.

Guillem, F., Bicu, M., Bloom, D. et al. (2001). Neuropsychological impairments in the syndromes of schizophrenia: a comparison between different dimensional models. *Brain and Cognition*, 46, 153–159.

Halligan, P. W., & David, A. S. (2001). Cognitive neuropsychiatry: towards a scientific psychopathology. *Nature Reviews Neuroscience*, 2, 209–215.

Halligan, P. W., & Marshall, J. C. (1995). Supernumerary phantom limb after right hemispheric stroke. *Journal of Neurology, Neurosurgery and Psychiatry*, 59, 341–342.

Halligan, P. W., Marshall, J. C., & Wade, D. T. (1993). Three arms: a case study of supernumerary phantom limb after right hemisphere stroke. *Journal of Neurology, Neurosurgery and Psychiatry*, 56, 159–166.

Harmon-Jones, E. & Mills, J. (Eds.). (1999) *Cognitive Dissonance: Progress on a Pivotal Theory in Social Psychology*. Washington, DC: American Psychological Association.

Hashimoto, R., Tanaka, Y., & Nakano, I. (2000). Amnesic confabulatory syndrome after focal basal forebrain damage. *Neurology*, 54, 978–980.

Hay, G. G. (1970). Dysmorphophobia. *British Journal of Psychiatry*, 116, 399–406.

Heilman, K. M. (1991). Anosognosia: possible neuropsychological mechanisms. In G. P. Prigatano & D. L. Schacter (Eds.), *Awareness of Deficit after Brain Injury* (pp. 53–62). New York/London: Oxford University Press.

Helmich, R. C., Hallett, M., Deuschl, G., Toni, I., & Bloem, B. R. (2012). Cerebral causes and consequences of Parkinsonian resting tremor: a tale of two circuits? *Brain*, 135, 3206–3226.

Helmsley, D. (1987). An experimental psychological model for schizophrenia. In H. Hafner, W. F. Gattaz & W. Janzarik (Eds.), *Search for the Causes of Schizophrenia* (pp.179–188). Berlin: Springer Verlag.

Hemsley, D. R., & Garety, P. A. (1986). The formation of maintenance of delusions: a Bayesian analysis. *British Journal of Psychiatry*, 149, 51–56.

Hietala, J., Syvalahti, E., Vuorio, K. et al. (1994). Striatal D2 dopamine receptor characteristics in neuroleptic-naive schizophrenic patients studied with positron emission tomography. *Archives of General Psychiatry*, 51, 116–123.

Himelhoch, S., Taylor, S. F., Goldman, R. S., & Tandon, R. (1996). Frontal lobe tasks, antipsychotic medication, and schizophrenia syndromes. *Biological Psychiatry*, 39, 227–229.

Hinzen, W., Rossello, J., & McKenna, P. (2016). Can delusions be understood linguistically? *Cognitive Neuropsychiatry*, 21, 281–299.

Hirstein, W., & Ramachandran, V. S. (1997). Capgras syndrome: a novel probe for understanding the neural representation of the identity and familiarity of persons. *Proceedings of the Royal Society B: Biological Sciences*, 264, 437–444.

Ho, D. Y. (1974). Modern logic and schizophrenic thinking. *Genetic Psychology Monographs*, 89, 145–165.

Hoch, P. H., & Polatin, P. (1949). Pseudoneurotic forms of schizophrenia. *Psychiatric Quarterly*, 33, 248–276.

Hodges, J. R. (Ed.). (2007). *Frontotemporal Dementia Syndromes*. Cambridge: Cambridge University Press.

Hodges, J. R., Patterson, K., Oxbury, S., & Funnell, E. (1992). Semantic dementia. Progressive fluent aphasia with temporal lobe atrophy. *Brain*, 115, 1783–1806.

Hofstadter, R. (1966). The paranoid style in American politics. In R. Hofstader (Ed.), *The Paranoid Style in American Politics and Other Essays* (pp. 3–40). New York: Knopf.

Hornykiewicz, O. (1976). Neurohumoral interactions and basal ganglia function and dysfunction. In M. D. Yahr (Ed.), *The Basal Ganglia*. New York: Raven Press.

House, A., & Hodges, J. (1988). Persistent denial of handicap after infarction of the right basal ganglia: a case study. *Journal of Neurology, Neurosurgery and Psychiatry*, 51, 112–115.

Howes, O. D., Montgomery, A. J., Asselin, M. C. et al. (2009). Elevated striatal dopamine function linked to prodromal signs of schizophrenia. *Archives of General Psychiatry*, 66, 13–20.

Howes, O. D., Bose, S. K., Turkheimer, F. et al. (2011a). Dopamine synthesis capacity before onset of psychosis: a prospective [18F]-DOPA PET imaging study. *American Journal of Psychiatry*, 168, 1311–1317.

Howes, O., Bose, S., Turkheimer, F. et al. (2011b). Progressive increase in striatal dopamine synthesis capacity as patients develop psychosis: a PET study. *Molecular Psychiatry*, 16, 885–886.

Hu, W., MacDonald, M. L., Elswick, D. E., & Sweet, R. A. (2015). The glutamate hypothesis of schizophrenia: evidence from human brain tissue studies. *Annals of the New York Academy of Sciences*, 1338, 38–57.

Huq, S. F., Garety, P. A., & Hemsley, D. R. (1988). Probabilistic judgements in deluded and non-deluded subjects. *Quarterly Journal of Experimental Psychology A*, 40, 801–812.

Insel, T. R., & Akiskal, H. S. (1986). Obsessive-compulsive disorder with psychotic features: a phenomenologic analysis. *American Journal of Psychiatry*, 143, 1527–1533.

Iversen, L. (2003). Cannabis and the brain. *Brain*, 126, 1252–1270.

Iversen, L. (2008a). *Speed, Ecstasy, Ritalin: The Science of Amphetamines*. Oxford: Oxford University Press.

Iversen, L. L. (2008b). *The Science of Marijuana*, 2nd Edition. Oxford: Oxford University Press.

Janis, I. L. (1983). *Groupthink: Psychological Studies of Policy Decisions and Fiascoes*, 2nd Edition. Boston: Houghton Mifflin.

Jaspers, K. (1912). The phenomenological approach in psychopathology. *Zeitschrift für die gesamte Neurologie und Psychiatrie*, 9, 391–408. Translated (1968). In *British Journal of Psychiatry*, 114, 1313–1323.

Jaspers, K. (1959). *General Psychopathology* (translated by J. Hoenig and M.W. Hamilton, 1963). Manchester: Manchester University Press.

Javitt, D. C., & Zukin, S. R. (1991). Recent advances in the phencyclidine model

of schizophrenia. *American Journal of Psychiatry*, 148, 1301–1308.

Jenkins, P. (1992). *Intimate Enemies: Moral Panics in Contemporary Great Britain*. New York: Aldine de Gruyter.

Johns, L. C. & van Os, J. (2001). The continuity of psychotic experiences in the general population. *Clinical Psychology Review*, 21, 1125–1141.

Johnstone, E. C., Crow, T. J., Frith, C. D., Husband, J., & Kreel, L. (1976). Cerebral ventricular size and cognitive impairment in chronic schizophrenia. *Lancet*, 2, 924–926.

Johnstone, M., Evans, V., & Baigel, S. (1959). Sernyl (CI-395) in clinical anaesthesia. *British Journal of Anaesthesia*, 31, 433–439.

Jones, E., & Watson, J. P. (1997). Delusion, the overvalued idea and religious beliefs: a comparative analysis of their characteristics. *British Journal of Psychiatry*, 170, 381–386.

Jones, H. (2003). In debate: Jaspers was right after all – delusions are distinct from normal beliefs. For. *British Journal of Psychiatry*, 183, 285.

Joyce, E. M., Collinson, S. L., & Crichton, P. (1996). Verbal fluency in schizophrenia: relationship with executive function, semantic memory and clinical alogia. *Psychological Medicine*, 26, 39–49.

Joyce, J. N. (1983). Multiple dopamine receptors and behavior. *Neuroscience and Biobehavioral Reviews*, 7, 227–256.

Kano, M. (2014). Control of synaptic function by endocannabinoid-mediated retrograde signaling. *Proceedings of the Japan Academy. Series B, Physical and Biological Sciences*, 90, 235–250.

Kano, M., Ohno-Shosaku, T., Hashimotodani, Y., Uchigashima, M., & Watanabe, M. (2009). Endocannabinoid-mediated control of synaptic transmission. *Physiological Reviews*, 89, 309–380.

Kapur, N., & Coughlan, A. K. (1980). Confabulation and frontal lobe dysfunction. *Journal of Neurology, Neurosurgery and Psychiatry*, 43, 461–463.

Kapur, N., Turner, A., & King, C. (1988). Reduplicative paramnesia: possible anatomical and neuropsychological mechanisms. *Journal of Neurology, Neurosurgery and Psychiatry*, 51, 579–581.

Kapur, S. (2003). Psychosis as a state of aberrant salience: a framework linking biology, phenomenology, and pharmacology in schizophrenia. *American Journal of Psychiatry*, 160, 13–23.

Kelley, A. E., & Domesick, V. B. (1982). The distribution of the projection from the hippocampal formation to the nucleus accumbens in the rat: an anterograde- and retrograde-horseradish peroxidase study. *Neuroscience*, 7, 2321–2335.

Kemp, R., Chua, S., McKenna, P., & David, A. (1997). Reasoning and delusions. *British Journal of Psychiatry*, 170, 398–405.

Kendler, K. S. (1980). The nosologic validity of paranoia (simple delusional disorder). A review. *Archives of General Psychiatry*, 37, 699–706.

Kendler, K. S. (1985). Diagnostic approaches to schizotypal personality disorder: a historical perspective. *Schizophrenia Bulletin*, 11, 538–553.

Kendler, K. S., Gallagher, T. J., Abelson, J. M., & Kessler, R. C. (1996). Lifetime prevalence, demographic risk factors, and diagnostic validity of nonaffective psychosis as assessed in a US community sample. The National Comorbidity Survey. *Archives of General Psychiatry*, 53, 1022–1031.

Kinon, B. J., Zhang, L., Millen, B. A. et al. (2011). a multicenter, inpatient, phase 2, double-blind, placebo-controlled dose-ranging study of LY2140023 monohydrate in patients with DSM-IV schizophrenia. *Journal of Clinical Psychopharmacology*, 31, 349–355.

Kintsch, W. (1980). Semantic memory: a tutorial. In R. S. Nickerson (Ed.), *Attention and Performance, VIII* (pp. 595–620). Hillsdale, NJ: Erlbaum.

Kipps, C. M., & Hodges, J. R. (2006). Theory of mind in frontotemporal dementia. *Society for Neuroscience*, 1, 235–244.

Knutson, B., Adams, C. M., Fong, G. W., & Hommer, D. (2001a). Anticipation of increasing monetary reward selectively recruits nucleus accumbens. *Journal of Neuroscience*, 21, RC159.

Knutson, B., Fong, G. W., Adams, C. M., Varner, J. L., & Hommer, D. (2001b). Dissociation of reward anticipation and outcome with event-related fMRI. *Neuroreport*, 12, 3683–3687.

Knutson, B., Taylor, J., Kaufman, M., Peterson, R., & Glover, G. (2005). Distributed neural representation of expected value. *Journal of Neuroscience*, 25, 4806–4812.

Knutson, B., Westdorp, A., Kaiser, E., & Hommer, D. (2000). FMRI visualization of brain activity during a monetary incentive delay task. *Neuroimage*, 12, 20–27.

Kolle, K. (1931). *Die primäre Verrücktheit*. Leipzig: Thieme.

Kopelman, M. D. (2010). Varieties of confabulation and delusion. *Cognitive Neuropsychiatry*, 15, 14–37.

Kovacs, M., & Beck, A. T. (1978). Maladaptive cognitive structures in depression. *American Journal of Psychiatry*, 135, 525–533.

Kozak, M. J., & Foa, E. B. (1994). Obsessions, overvalued ideas, and delusions in obsessive-compulsive disorder. *Behaviour Research and Therapy*, 32, 343–353.

Kraepelin, E. (1905). *Lectures on Clinical Psychiatry*, 3rd English Edition, *(translated by T. Johnstone, 1917)*. New York: W. Wood.

Kraepelin, E. (1907). *Clinical Psychiatry*, 7th edition (translated by A. R. Diefendorf). London: MacMillan.

Kraepelin, E. (1913a). *Dementia Praecox and Paraphrenia* (translated by R. M. Barclay, 1919). Edinburgh: Livingstone.

Kraepelin, E. (1913b). *Manic-Depressive Insanity and Paranoia* (translated by R. M. Barclay, 1921). Edinburgh: Livingstone.

Kreiskott, H. (1980). Behavioral pharmacology of antipsychotics. In F. Hoffmeister & G. Stille (Eds.), *Handbook of Experimental Pharmacology, Volume 55, Psychotropic Agents. Part 1: Antipsychotics and Antidepressants* (pp. 59–88). Berlin: Springer.

Kreitzer, A. C. & Regehr, W. G. (2001). Cerebellar depolarization-induced suppression of inhibition is mediated by endogenous cannabinoids. *Journal of Neuroscience*, 21, RC174.

Kretschmer, E. (1927). The sensitive delusion of reference. Translated (1974). In S. R. Hirsch & M. Shepherd (Eds.), *Themes and Variations in European Psychiatry* (pp. 153–195). Bristol: Wright.

Krystal, J. H., Karper, L. P., Seibyl, J. P. et al. (1994). Subanesthetic effects of the noncompetitive nmda antagonist, ketamine, in humans. Psychotomimetic, perceptual, cognitive, and neuroendocrine responses. *Archives of General Psychiatry*, 51, 199–214.

Kuczenski, R., & Segal, D. S. (1997). Effects of methylphenidate on extracellular dopamine, serotonin, and norepinephrine: comparison with amphetamine. *Journal of Neurochemistry*, 68, 2032–2037.

Kwapil, T. R., & Barrantes-Vidal, N. (2012). Schizotypal personality disorder: an integrative review. In T. A. Widiger (Ed.), *Oxford Handbook of Personality Disorders* (pp. 437–477). Oxford/New York Oxford University Press.

La Fontaine, J. S. (1998). *Speak of the Devil: Tales of Satanic Abuse in Contemporary England*. Cambridge: Cambridge University Press.

Lahti, A. C., Weiler, M. A., Tamara Michaelidis, B. A., Parwani, A., & Tamminga, C. A. (2001). Effects of ketamine in normal and schizophrenic volunteers. *Neuropsychopharmacology*, 25, 455–467.

Landin-Romero, R., McKenna, P. J., Romaguera, A. et al. (2016). Examining the continuum of psychosis: frequency and characteristics of psychotic-like symptoms in relatives and non-relatives of patients with schizophrenia. *Schizophrenia Research*, 178, 6–11.

Langdon, R., & Bayne, T. (2010). Delusion and confabulation: mistakes of perceiving, remembering and believing. *Cognitive Neuropsychiatry*, 15, 319–345.

Langdon, R., & Coltheart, M. (2000). The cognitive neuropsychology of delusions. *Mind and Language*, 15, 184–121.

Langdon, R., Ward, P. B., & Coltheart, M. (2010). Reasoning anomalies associated with delusions in schizophrenia. *Schizophrenia Bulletin*, 36, 321–330.

Laruelle, M., Abi-Dargham, A., Gil, R., Kegeles, L., & Innis, R. (1999). Increased dopamine transmission in schizophrenia: relationship to illness phases. *Biological Psychiatry*, 46, 56–72.

Laruelle, M., Abi-Dargham, A., van Dyck, C. H. et al. (1996). Single photon emission computerized tomography imaging of amphetamine-induced dopamine release in drug-free schizophrenic subjects. *Proceedings of the National Academy of Sciences USA*, 93, 9235–9240.

Laws, K. R., McKenna, P. J., & McCarthy, R. A. (1995). Delusions about people. *Neurocase*, 1, 349–362.

Lebert, F., Pasquier, F., Steinling, M. et al. (1994). SPECT data in a case of secondary Capgras delusion. *Psychopathology*, 27, 211–214.

LeBoeuf, R. A., & Norton, M. I. (2012). Consequence-cause matching: looking to the consequences of events to infer their causes. *Journal of Consumer Research*, 39, 128–141.

Leman, P. J., & Cinnirella, M. (2007). A major event has a major cause. *Social Psychological Review*, 9, 18–28.

Lenzenweger, M. F. (2010). *Schizotypy and Schizophrenia: The View from Experimental Psychology*. New York/London: Guildford.

Lewis, A. J. (1934). Melancholia: a clinical survey of depressive states. *Journal of Mental Science*, 277–378. Reprinted in A. Lewis (Ed.) (1967), *Inquiries in Psychiatry: Clinical and Social Investigations* (pp. 30–117). London: Routledge and Kegan Paul, 1967.

Lewis, A. (1936). Problems of obsessional illness. *Proceedings of the Royal Society of Medicine*, 29, 325–336. Reprinted in A. Lewis (Ed.) (1967), *Inquiries in Psychiatry: Clinical and Social Investigations* (pp. 141–156). London: Routledge and Kegan Paul.

Lewis, A. (1957). Obsessional illness. *Acta Neuropsiquiátrica Argentina*, 3, 323–335. Reprinted in A. Lewis (Ed.) (1967), *Inquiries in Psychiatry: Clinical and Social Investigations* (pp. 157–172). London: Routledge and Kegan Paul.

Liddle, P. F. (1987a). The symptoms of chronic schizophrenia. A re-examination of the positive-negative dichotomy. *British Journal of Psychiatry*, 151, 145–151.

Liddle, P. F. (1987b). Schizophrenic syndromes, cognitive performance and neurological dysfunction. *Psychological Medicine*, 17, 49–57.

Liddle, P. F., & Morris, D. L. (1991). Schizophrenic syndromes and frontal lobe performance. *British Journal of Psychiatry*, 158, 340–345.

Lincoln, T. M., Ziegler, M., Mehl, S., & Rief, W. (2010). The jumping to conclusions bias in delusions: specificity and changeability. *Journal of Abnormal Psychology*, 119, 40–49.

Lindstrom, L. (1993). *Cargo Cult: Strange Stories of Desire from Melanesia and Beyond.* Honolulu: University of Hawaii Press.

Linscott, R. J. & van Os, J. (2013). An updated and conservative systematic review and meta-analysis of epidemiological evidence on psychotic experiences in children and adults: on the pathway from proneness to persistence to dimensional expression across mental disorders. *Psychological Medicine*, 43, 1133–1149.

Lishman, W. A. (1998). *Organic Psychiatry*, 3rd Edition. Oxford: Blackwell Science.

Lord, C. G., Ross, L., & Lepper, M. R. (1979). Biased assimilation and attitude polarization: the effects of prior theories on subsequently considered evidence. *Journal of Personality and Social Psychology*, 37, 2098–2109.

Luby, E. D., Cohen, B. D., Rosenbaum, G., Gottlieb, J. S., & Kelley, R. (1959). Study of a new schizophrenomimetic drug – sernyl. *A.M.A. Archives of Neurology and Psychiatry*, 81, 363–369.

Lucas, A. R., & Weiss, M. (1971). Methylphenidate hallucinosis. *Journal of the American Medical Association*, 217, 1079–1081.

Lunt, L., Bramham, J., Morris, R. G. et al. (2012). Prefrontal cortex dysfunction and 'Jumping to Conclusions': bias or deficit? *Journal of Neuropsychology*, 6, 65–78.

MacCallum, W. A. (1973). Capgras symptoms with an organic basis. *British Journal of Psychiatry*, 123, 639–642.

Maher, B. A. (1974). Delusional thinking and perceptual disorder. *Journal of Individual Psychology*, 30, 98–113.

Maher, B., & Ross, J. S. (1984). Delusions. In H. E. Adams & P. B. Sutker (Eds.), *Comprehensive Handbook of Psychopathology* (pp. 383–409). New York: Plenum.

Maina, G., Albert, U., Bada, A., & Bogetto, F. (2001). Occurrence and clinical correlates of psychiatric co-morbidity in delusional disorder. *European Psychiatry*, 16, 222–228.

Malenka, R. C., & Bear, M. F. (2004). LTP and LTD: an embarrassment of riches. *Neuron*, 44, 5–21.

Marneros, A. (2012). *Persistent Delusional Disorders: Myths and Realities.* New York: Nova.

Marneros, A., Pillmann, F., & Wustmann, T. (2012). Delusional disorders – are they simply paranoid schizophrenia? *Schizophrenia Bulletin*, 38, 561–568.

Martin, S. J., Grimwood, P. D., & Morris, R. G. (2000). Synaptic plasticity and memory: an evaluation of the hypothesis. *Annual Review of Neuroscience*, 23, 649–711.

Martinot, J. L., Peron-Magnan, P., Huret, J. D. et al. (1990). Striatal D2 dopaminergic receptors assessed with positron emission tomography and [76Br]bromospiperone in untreated schizophrenic patients. *American Journal of Psychiatry*, 147, 44–50.

Mason, S. T. (1984). *Catecholamines and Behaviour.* Cambridge: Cambridge University Press.

Matsuda, W., Furuta, T., Nakamura, K. C. et al. (2009). Single nigrostriatal dopaminergic neurons form widely spread and highly dense axonal arborizations in the neostriatum. *Journal of Neuroscience*, 29, 444–453.

Mattioli, F., Miozzo, A., & Vignolo, L. A. (1999). Confabulation and delusional misidentification: a four year follow-up study. *Cortex*, 35, 413–422.

McCarron, M. M., Schulze, B. W., Thompson, G. A., Conder, M. C., & Goetz, W. A. (1981). Acute phencyclidine intoxication: clinical patterns, complications, and treatment. *Annals of Emergency Medicine*, 10, 290–297.

McCauley, C., & Jacques, S. (1979). Popularity of conspiracy theories of presidential assassination: a Bayesian analysis. *Journal of Personality and Social Psychology*, 37, 637–644.

McClure, S. M., York, M. K., & Montague, P. R. (2004). The neural substrates of reward processing in humans: the modern role of FMRI. *The Neuroscientist*, 10, 260–268.

McDonald, N. (1960). Living with schizophrenia. *Canadian Medical Association Journal*, 82, 218–221.

McGhie, A., & Chapman, J. (1961). Disorders of attention and perception in early schizophrenia. *British Journal of Medical Psychology*, 34, 103–116.

McGrath, J. (1991). Ordering thoughts on thought disorder. *British Journal of Psychiatry*, 158, 307–316.

McKenna, P. J. (1984). Disorders with overvalued ideas. *British Journal of Psychiatry*, 145, 579–585.

McKenna, P. J. (1987). Pathology, phenomenology and the dopamine hypothesis of schizophrenia. *British Journal of Psychiatry*, 151, 288–301.

McKenna, P. J. (1991). Memory, knowledge and delusions. *British Journal of Psychiatry Supplement*, 14, 36–41.

McKenna, P. J. (1994). *Schizophrenia and Related Syndromes*. Oxford: Oxford University Press.

McKenna, P. J. (2007). *Schizophrenia and Related Syndromes, 2nd edition*. Hove, Sussex: Routledge.

McKenna, P. J., & Oh, T. (2005). *Schizophrenic Speech: Making Sense of Bathroots and Ponds That Fall in Doorways*. Cambridge: Cambridge University Press.

Meehl, P. E. (1962). Schizotaxia, schizotypy, schizophrenia. *American Psychologist*, 17, 827–838.

Menon, M., Pomarol-Clotet, E., McKenna, P. J., & McCarthy, R. A. (2006). Probabilistic reasoning in schizophrenia: a comparison of the performance of deluded and nondeluded schizophrenic patients and exploration of possible cognitive underpinnings. *Cognitive Neuropsychiatry*, 11, 521–536.

Mercer, B., Wapner, W., Gardner, H., & Benson, D. F. (1977). A study of confabulation. *Archives of Neurology*, 34, 429–433.

Merskey, H. (1979). *The Analysis of Hysteria*. London/Sydney: Baillière Tindall.

Metcalf, K., Langdon, R., & Coltheart, M. (2007). Models of confabulation: a critical review and a new framework. *Cognitive Neuropsychology*, 24, 23–47.

Miller, R. (1984). Major psychosis and dopamine: controversial features and some suggestions. *Psychological Medicine*, 14, 779–789.

Millon, T., Grossman, S., Meagher, S., & Ramnath, R. (2004). *Personality Disorders in Modern Life*, 2nd Edition. Hoboken, NJ: Wiley.

Mohamed, S., Paulsen, J. S., O'Leary, D., Arndt, S., & Andreasen, N. (1999). Generalized cognitive deficits in schizophrenia: a study of first-episode patients. *Archives of General Psychiatry*, 56, 749–754.

Monbiot, G. (2007). Short changed. Retrieved 12 February 2007, from www.monbiot.com/2007/02/12/short-changed/.

Montag, C., Dziobek, I., Richter, I. S. et al. (2011). Different aspects of theory of mind in paranoid schizophrenia: evidence from a video-based assessment. *Psychiatry Research*, 186, 203–209.

Moore, T. H., Zammit, S., Lingford-Hughes, A. et al. (2007). Cannabis use and risk of psychotic or affective mental health outcomes: a systematic review. *Lancet*, 370, 319–328.

Moreau, J. J. (1845). *Du Haschisch et de l'alienation Mentale* (Translated 1973 as *Hashish and Mental Illness* by Peters, H. and Nahas, G.). New York: Raven.

Moritz, S., & Woodward, T. S. (2005). Jumping to conclusions in delusional and non-delusional schizophrenic patients. *British Journal of Clinical Psychology*, 44, 193–207.

Moritz, S., Andresen, B., Jacobsen, D. et al. (2001). Neuropsychological correlates of schizophrenic syndromes in patients treated with atypical neuroleptics. *European Psychiatry*, 16, 354–361.

Mortimer, A. M., Bentham, P., McKay, A. P. et al. (1996). Delusions in schizophrenia: a phenomenological and psychological exploration. *Cognitive Neuropsychiatry*, 1, 289–304.

Moscovitch, M. (1992). Memory and working-with-memory: a component process model based on modules and central systems. *Journal of Cognitive Neuroscience*, 4, 257–267.

Moscovitch, M. (1995). Confabulation. In D. L. Schacter (Ed.), *Memory Distortion: How Minds, Brains, and Societies Reconstruct the Past* (pp. 226–251). Cambridge, MA/London: Harvard University Press.

Moscovitch, M., & Melo, B. (1997). Strategic retrieval and the frontal lobes: evidence from confabulation and amnesia. *Neuropsychologia*, 35, 1017–1034.

Mosholder, A. D., Gelperin, K., Hammad, T. A., Phelan, K., & Johann-Liang, R. (2009). Hallucinations and other psychotic symptoms associated with the use of attention-deficit/hyperactivity disorder drugs in children. *Pediatrics*, 123, 611–616.

Mullen, P. E., Pathé, M., & Purcell, R. (2000). *Stalkers and Their Victims*. Cambridge: Cambridge University Press.

Munro, A. (1978). Monosymptomatic hypochondriacal psychoses: a diagnostic entity which may respond to pimozide. *Canadian Psychiatric Association Journal*, 23, 497–500.

Munro, A. (1980). Monosymptomatic hypochondriacal psychosis. *British Journal of Hospital Medicine*, 24, 34, 36–38.

Munro, A. (1982). Delusional hypochondriasis. *Clarke Institute of Psychiatry Monograph no. 5* Toronto: Clarke Institute of Psychiatry.

Munro, A. (1988). Monosymptomatic hypochondriacal psychosis. *British Journal of Psychiatry Supplement*, 2, 37–40.

Munro, A. (1999). *Delusional Disorder: Paranoia and Related Illnesses*. Cambridge: Cambridge University Press.

Munro, A., & Chmara, J. (1982). Monosymptomatic hypochondriacal psychosis: a diagnostic checklist based on 50 cases of the disorder. *Canadian Journal of Psychiatry*, 27, 374–376.

Murray, G. K., Corlett, P. R., Clark, L. et al. (2008). Substantia nigra/ventral tegmental reward prediction error disruption in psychosis. *Molecular Psychiatry*, 13, 239, 267–276.

Nathan, D. (2001). *Satan's Silence: Ritual Abuse and the Making af a Modern American Witch Hunt*. Bloomington, IN: iUniverse.

Nathanson, M., Bergman, P. S., & Gordon, G. G. (1952). Denial of illness; its occurrence in one hundred consecutive cases of hemiplegia. *AMA Archives of Neurology and Psychiatry*, 68, 380–387.

Newcomer, J. W., Farber, N. B., Jevtovic-Todorovic, V. et al. (1999). Ketamine-induced NMDA receptor hypofunction as a model of memory impairment and psychosis. *Neuropsychopharmacology*, 20, 106–118.

Norman, R. M., Malla, A. K., Morrison-Stewart, S. L. et al. (1997). Neuropsychological correlates of syndromes in schizophrenia. *British Journal of Psychiatry*, 170, 134–139.

Ochoa, S., Haro, J. M., Huerta-Ramos, E. et al. (2014). Relation between jumping to conclusions and cognitive functioning in people with schizophrenia in contrast with healthy participants. *Schizophr Research*, 159, 211–217.

O'Dwyer, A. M., & Marks, I. (2000). Obsessive-compulsive disorder and delusions revisited. *British Journal of Psychiatry*, 176, 281–284.

O'Keefe, J., & Nadel, L. (1978). *The Hippocampus as a Cognitive Map*. Oxford: Clarendon Press.

Olds, J., & Milner, P. (1954). Positive reinforcement produced by electrical stimulation of septal area and other regions of rat brain. *Journal of Comparative and Physiological Psychology*, 47, 419–427.

O'Leary, D. S., Flaum, M., Kesler, M. L. et al. (2000). Cognitive correlates of the negative, disorganized, and psychotic symptom dimensions of schizophrenia. *Journal of Neuropsychiatry and Clinical Neuroscience*, 12, 4–15.

Ormrod, J., Shaftoe, D., Cavanagh, K. et al. (2012). A pilot study exploring the contribution of working memory to 'jumping to conclusions' in people with first episode psychosis. *Cognitive Neuropsychiatry*, 17, 97–114.

Park, W.-W. (1990). A review of research on groupthink. *Journal of Behavioral Decision Making*, 3, 229–245.

Patil, S. T., Zhang, L., Martenyi, F. et al. (2007). Activation of Mglu2/3 receptors as a new approach to treat schizophrenia: a randomized phase 2 clinical trial. *Nature Medicine*, 13, 1102–1107.

Pavlac, B. A. (2009). *Witch Hunts in the Western World. Persecution and Punishment from the Inquisition through the Salem Trials*. Lincoln, NE: University of Nebraska Press.

Peralta, V., & Cuesta, M. J. (1994). Psychometric properties of the positive and negative syndrome scale (PANSS) in schizophrenia. *Psychiatry Research*, 53, 31–40.

Peters, E. R., Joseph, S. A., & Garety, P. A. (1999). Measurement of delusional ideation in the normal population: introducing the PDI (Peters et al. Delusions Inventory). *Schizophrenia Bulletin*, 25, 553–576.

Peters, E. R., Thornton, P., Siksou, L., Linney, Y., & MacCabe, J. H. (2008). Specificity of the jump-to-conclusions bias in deluded patients. *British Journal of Clinical Psychology*, 47, 239–244.

Phillips, K. A. (2004). Psychosis in body dysmorphic disorder. *Journal of Psychiatric Research*, 38, 63–72.

Phillips, K. A. (2005a). *The Broken Mirror: Understanding and Treating Body Dysmorphic Disorder*, revised and expanded edition. Oxford/New York: Oxford University Press.

Phillips, K. A. (2005b). Placebo-controlled study of pimozide augmentation of fluoxetine in body dysmorphic disorder. *American Journal of Psychiatry*, 162, 377–379.

Phillips, K. A., McElroy, S. L., Keck, P. E., Jr., Hudson, J. I., & Pope, H. G., Jr. (1994). A comparison of delusional and nondelusional body dysmorphic disorder in 100 cases. *Psychopharmacology Bulletin*, 30, 179–186.

Phillips, K. A., Menard, W., Pagano, M. E., Fay, C., & Stout, R. L. (2006). Delusional versus nondelusional body dysmorphic disorder: clinical features and course of illness. *Journal of Psychiatric Research*, 40, 95–104.

Pilowsky, L. S., Costa, D. C., Ell, P. J. et al. (1994). D2 dopamine receptor binding in the basal ganglia of antipsychotic-free schizophrenic patients. An 123I-IBZM single photon emission computerised tomography study. *British Journal of Psychiatry*, 164, 16–26.

Pollice, R., Roncone, R., Falloon, I. R. et al. (2002). Is theory of mind in schizophrenia more strongly associated with clinical and social functioning than with neurocognitive deficits? *Psychopathology*, 35, 280–288.

Pomarol-Clotet, E., Honey, G. D., Murray, G. K. et al. (2006). Psychological effects of ketamine in healthy volunteers. Phenomenological study. *British Journal of Psychiatry*, 189, 173–179.

Radhakrishnan, R., Wilkinson, S. T., & D'Souza, D. C. (2014). Gone to pot – a review of the association between cannabis and psychosis. *Frontiers in Psychiatry*, 5, 54.

Radua, J., Schmidt, A., Borgwardt, S. et al. (2015). Ventral striatal activation during reward processing in psychosis: a neurofunctional meta-analysis. *JAMA Psychiatry*, 72, 1243–1251.

Raffaele, P. (2006). In John they trust. *Smithsonian Magazine*, February, 2006. (www.smithsonianmag.com/people-places/in-john-they-trust-109294882/?page=1%3Fno-ist), last accessed 28 March 2017.

Ramachandran, V. S. (1996). What neurological syndromes can tell us about human nature: some lessons from phantom limbs, capgras syndrome, and anosognosia. *Cold Spring Harbor Symposia on Quantitative Biology*, 61, 115–134.

Rescorla, R. A., & Wagner, A. R. (1972). A theory of Pavlovian conditioning: variations in the effectiveness of reinforcement and nonreinforcement. In A. H. Black & W. F. Prokasy (Eds.), *Classical Conditioning II: Current Research and Theory* (pp. 64–99). New York: Appleton Century Crofts.

Riding, J., & Munro, A. (1975a). Pimozide in the treatment of monosymptomatic hypochondriacal psychosis. *Acta Psychiatrica Scandinavica*, 52, 23–30.

Riding, B. E., & Munro, A. (1975b). Letter: Pimozide in monosymptomatic psychosis. *Lancet*, 1, 400–401.

Robbins, T. W. (1990). The case of frontostriatal dysfunction in schizophrenia. *Schizophrenia Bulletin*, 16, 391–402.

Robbins, T. W., & Everitt, B. J. (1992). Functions of dopamine in the dorsal and ventral striatum. *Seminars in Neuroscience* 4, 119–127.

Robert, P. H., Lafont, V., Medecin, I. et al. (1998). Clustering and switching strategies in verbal fluency tasks: comparison between schizophrenics and healthy adults. *Journal of the International Neuropsychological Society*, 4, 539–546.

Roberts, J., & Roberts, R. (1977). Delusions of parasitosis. *British Medical Journal*, i, 1219.

Robins, L. N., Cottler, L. B., Bucholz, K. K. et al. (2000). *Computerized Diagnostic Interview Schedule for the DSM-IV (C DIS-IV)*: NIMH/ University of Florida.

Robinson, S., Winnik, H. Z., & Weiss, A. A. (1976). 'Obsessive psychosis': justification for a separate clinical entity. *Israel Annals of Psychiatry and Related Disciplines*, 14, 39–48.

Rodriguez-Oroz, M. C., Jahanshahi, M., Krack, P. et al. (2009). Initial clinical manifestations of Parkinson's disease: features and pathophysiological mechanisms. *Lancet Neurology*, 8, 1128–1139.

Ron, M. A., & Logsdail, S. J. (1989). Psychiatric morbidity in multiple sclerosis: a clinical and MRI study. *Psychological Medicine*, 19, 887–895.

Rosen, I. (1957). The clinical significance of obsessions in schizophrenia. *Journal of Mental Science*, 103, 773–785.

Rossell, S. L., Shapleske, J., & David, A. S. (1998). Sentence verification and delusions: a content-specific deficit. *Psychological Medicine*, 28, 1189–1198.

Rowe, E. W., & Shean, G. (1997). Card-sort performance and syndromes of schizophrenia. *Genetic, Social and General Psychology Monographs*, 123, 197–209.

Ruitenberg, M. F., Duthoo, W., Santens, P., Notebaert, W., & Abrahamse, E. L. (2015). Sequential movement skill in Parkinson's disease: a state-of-the-art. *Cortex*, 65, 102–112.

Rylander, G. (1972). Psychoses and the punding and choreiform syndromes in addiction to central stimulant drugs. *Psychiatria, Neurologia, Neurochirurgia*, 75, 203–212.

Sandifer, P. H. (1946). Anosognosia and disorders of body scheme. *Brain*, 69, 122–137.

Schiorring, E. (1981). Psychopathology induced by 'speed drugs'. *Pharmacology, Biochemistry, and Behavior*, 14 Suppl 1, 109–122.

Schneider, K. (1930). *Psychologie der Schizophrenen*. Leipzig: Thieme.

Schneider, K. (1949). The concept of delusion. Translated (1974). In S. R. Hirsch & M. Shepherd (Eds.), *Themes and Variations in European Psychiatry* (pp. 33–39). Bristol: Wright.

Schneider, K. (1958). *Clinical Psychopathology*, 5th edition (translated (1959) by M.W. Hamilton). New York: Grune and Stratton.

Schultz, W. (1998). Predictive reward signal of dopamine neurons. *Journal of Neurophysiology*, 80, 1–27.

Seeman, P. (1987). Dopamine receptors and the dopamine hypothesis of schizophrenia. *Synapse*, 1, 133–152.

Seger, C. A. (2006). The basal ganglia in human learning. *The Neuroscientist*, 12, 285–290.

Seidman, L. J. (1983). Schizophrenia and brain dysfunction: an integration of recent neurodiagnostic findings. *Psychological Bulletin*, 94, 195–238.

Shakeel, M. K., & Docherty, N. M. (2015). Confabulations in schizophrenia. *Cognitive Neuropsychiatry*, 20, 1–13.

Shallice, T., Burgess, P. W., & Frith, C. D. (1991). Can the neuropsychological case-study approach be applied to schizophrenia? *Psychological Medicine*, 21, 661–673.

Shorter, E. (1997). *A History of Psychiatry: From the Era of the Asylum to the Age of Prozac*. New York: Wiley.

Sidgwick, H., Johnson, A., Myers, F. W. H., Podmore, F., & Sidgwick, E. (1894). Report on the census of hallucinations. In *Proceedings of the Society for Psychical Research*, Vol XXVI, part X. London: Kegan Paul, Trench Trübner.

Signer, S. F. (1991). De Clérambault's concept of erotomania and its place in his thought. *History of Psychiatry*, 2, 409–417.

Sims, A. (1988). *Symptoms in the Mind: An Introduction to Descriptive Psychopathology*. London: W. B. Saunders.

Sims, A. (1995). *Symptoms in the Mind: An Introduction to Descriptive Psychopathology*, 2nd Edition. London: W. B. Saunders.

Skott, A. (1978). Delusions of Infestation. Dermatozoenwahn – Ekbom's Syndrome. Reports from the Psychiatric Research Centre, St Jorgen Hospital, no. 13. Goteberg, Sweden: University of Goteberg.

Snowden, J. S., Goulding, P. J., & Neary, D. (1989). Semantic dementia: a form of circumscribed cerebral atrophy. *Behavioural Neurology*, 2, 167–182.

Snowden, J. S., Neary, D., & Mann, D. M. A. (1996). *Fronto-Temporal Lobar Degeneration: Fronto-Temporal Dementia, Progressive Aphasia, Semantic Dementia*. New York: Churchill Livingstone.

So, S. H., Freeman, D., Dunn, G. et al. (2012). Jumping to conclusions, a lack of belief flexibility and delusional conviction in psychosis: a longitudinal investigation of the structure, frequency, and relatedness of reasoning biases. *Journal of Abnormal Psychology*, 121, 129–139.

Solyom, L., DiNicola, V. F., Phil, M., Sookman, D., & Luchins, D. (1985). Is there an obsessive psychosis? Aetiological and prognostic factors of an atypical form of obsessive-compulsive neurosis. *Canadian Journal of Psychiatry*, 30, 372–380.

Spitzer, R. L., Gibbon, M., Skodol, A. E., Williams, J. B. W., & First, M. B. (1989). *DSM-III-R Case Book*. Washington, DC: American Psychiatric Press.

Spitzer, R. L., Gibbon, M., Skodol, A. E., Williams, J. B. W., & First, M. B. (1994). *DSM-IV Case Book*. Washington, DC: American Psychiatric Press.

Sprong, M., Schothorst, P., Vos, E., Hox, J., & van Engeland, H. (2007). Theory of mind in schizophrenia: meta-analysis. *British Journal of Psychiatry*, 191, 5–13.

Staton, R. D., Brumback, R. A., & Wilson, H. (1982). Reduplicative paramnesia: a disconnection syndrome of memory. *Cortex*, 18, 23–35.

Stengel, E. (1945). A study on some clinical aspects of the relationship between obsessional neurosis and psychotic reaction types. *Journal of Mental Science*, 91, 166–187.

Stone, T., & Young, A. W. (1997). Delusions and brain injury: the philosophy and psychology of belief. *Mind and Language*, 12, 327–364.

Storm-Mathisen, J. (1981). Glutamate in hippocampal pathways. *Advances in Biochemical Psychopharmacology*, 27, 43–55.

Stuss, D. T., Alexander, M. P., Lieberman, A., & Levine, H. (1978). An extraordinary form of confabulation. *Neurology*, 28, 1166–1172.

Sutherland, S. (1992). *Irrationality: The Enemy Within*. London: Constable and Company.

Swami, S. & Rebecca Coles, R. (2010). The truth is out there. *The Psychologist*, 23, 560–563.

Tabares, R., Sanjuan, J., Gomez-Beneyto, M., & Leal, C. (2000). Correlates of symptom dimensions in schizophrenia obtained with the Spanish version of the Manchester scale. *Psychopathology*, 33, 259–264.

Takeuchi, T., Duszkiewicz, A. J., & Morris, R. G. (2014). The synaptic plasticity and memory hypothesis: encoding, storage and persistence. *Philosophical Transactions of the Royal Society of London. Series B, Biological Sciences*, 369, 20130288.

Tamlyn, D., McKenna, P. J., Mortimer, A. M. et al. (1992). Memory impairment in schizophrenia: its extent, affiliations and neuropsychological character. *Psychological Medicine*, 22, 101–115.

Tatetsu, S. (1964). Methamphetamine psychosis. *Folia Psychiatrica et Neurologica Japonica*, Supplement 7, 377–380.

Thomas, H. (1993). Psychiatric symptoms in cannabis users. *British Journal of Psychiatry*, 163, 141–149.

Thompson, P. A., & Meltzer, H. Y. (1993). Positive, negative, and disorganisation factors from the Schedule for Affective Disorders and Schizophrenia and the Present State Examination. A three-factor solution. *British Journal of Psychiatry*, 163, 344–351.

Tranel, D., Damasio, H., & Damasio, A. R. (1995). Double dissociation between overt and covert face recognition. *Journal of Cognitive Neuroscience*, 7, 425–432.

Tulving, E. (1972). Episodic and semantic memory. In E. Tulving & W. Donaldson

(Eds.), *Organization of Memory* (pp 382–403). New York: Academic Press.

Tulving, E. (1983). *Elements of Episodic Memory.* Oxford: Clarendon Press.

Tuominen, H. J., Tiihonen, J., & Wahlbeck, K. (2005). Glutamatergic drugs for schizophrenia: a systematic review and meta-analysis. *Schizophrenia Research*, 72, 225–234.

Turner, M. S., Cipolotti, L., Yousry, T. A., & Shallice T. (2008). Confabulation: damage to a specific inferior medial prefrontal system. *Cortex*, 44, 637–648.

Turner, M., & Coltheart, M. (2010). Confabulation and delusion: a common monitoring framework. *Cognitive Neuropsychiatry* , 15, 346–376.

Tversky, A., & Kahneman, D. (1974). Judgment under uncertainty: heuristics and biases. *Science*, 185, 1124–1131.

Ullman, M. (1962). *Behavioral Changes in Patients following Stroke.* Springfield, IL: Charles C. Thomas.

Van der Does, A. J., Dingemans, P. M., Linszen, D. H., Nugter, M. A., & Scholte, W. F. (1993). Symptom dimensions and cognitive and social functioning in recent-onset schizophrenia. *Psychological Medicine*, 23, 745–753.

van Os, J. (2009). 'Salience syndrome' replaces 'schizophrenia' in DSM-V and ICD-11: psychiatry's evidence-based entry into the 21st century? *Acta Psychiatrica Scandinavica*, 120, 363–372.

van Os, J., Hanssen, M., Bijl, R. V., & Ravelli, A. (2000). Strauss (1969) revisited: a psychosis continuum in the general population? *Schizophrenia Research*, 45, 11–20.

van Os, J., Linscott, R. J., Myin-Germeys, I., Delespaul, P., & Krabbendam, L. (2009). A systematic review and meta-analysis of the psychosis continuum: evidence for a psychosis proneness-persistence-impairment model of psychotic disorder. *Psychological Medicine*, 39, 179–195.

Veale, D. (2002). Over-valued ideas: a conceptual analysis. *Behaviour Research and Therapy*, 40, 383–400.

Ventura, J., Wood, R. C., & Hellemann, G. S. (2013). Symptom domains and neurocognitive functioning can help differentiate social cognitive processes in schizophrenia: a meta-analysis. *Schizophrenia Bulletin*, 39, 102–111.

Verdoux, H., Maurice-Tison, S., Gay, B. et al. (1998). A survey of delusional ideation in primary-care patients. *Psychological Medicine*, 28, 127–134.

Vicens, V., Sarro, S., & McKenna, P. J. (2011). Comorbidity of delusional disorder with bipolar disorder: report of four cases. *Journal of Affective Disorders*, 134, 431–433.

Victor, J. S. (1993). *Satanic Panic: The Creation of a Contemporary Legend.* Chicago: Open Court Publishing Company.

Volans, P. J. (1976). Styles of decision-making and probability appraisal in selected obsessional and phobic patients. *British Journal of Social and Clinical Psychology*, 15, 305–317.

von Domarus, E. (1944). The specific laws of logic in schizophrenia. In J. S. Kasanin (Ed.), *Language and Thought in Schizophrenia* (pp. 104–114). New York: W.W. Norton.

Walker, C. (1991). Delusion: what did Jaspers really say? *British Journal of Psychiatry*, 159, Supplement 14, 94–101.

Walston, F., Blennerhassett, R. C., & Charlton, B. C. (2000). 'Theory of mind', persecutory delusions and the somatic marker mechanism. *Cognitive Neuropsychiatry*, 5, 161–174.

Warrington, E. K. (1975). The selective impairment of semantic memory. *Quarterly Journal of Experimental Psychology*, 27, 635–657.

Watson, C. G., Wold, J., & Kucala, T. (1976). A comparison of abstractive and nonabstractive deficits in schizophrenics and psychiatric controls. *Journal of Nervous and Mental Disease*, 163, 193–199.

Watson, C. G., & Wold, J. (1981). Logical reasoning deficits in schizophrenia and brain damage. *Journal of Clinical Psychology*, 37, 466–471.

Weinberger, D. R. (1988). Schizophrenia and the frontal lobe. *Trends in Neurosciences*, 11, 367–370.

Weinstein, E. (1970). Woodrow Wilson's neurological illness. *Journal of American History*, 57, 324–351.

Weinstein, E. A. (1969). Patterns of reduplication in organic brain disease. In P. J. Vinken & G. W. Bruyn (Eds.), *Handbook of Clinical Neurology, Volume 3* (pp. 251–257). Amsterdam: North Holland Publishing Company.

Weinstein, E. A. (1994). The classification of delusional misidentification syndromes. *Psychopathology*, 27, 130–135.

Weinstein, E. A., & Kahn, R. L. (1950). The syndrome of anosognosia. *AMA Archives of Neurology and Psychiatry*, 64, 772–791.

Weinstein, E. A., & Kahn, R. L. (1955). *Denial of Illness*. Springfield, IL: Charles C. Thomas.

Wernicke, C. (1906). *Grundriss der Psychiatrie in klinischen Vorlesungen, Zweite revidierte Auflage*. Leipzig: Verlag von Georg Thieme. Translated 2015 as *An Outline of Psychiatry in Clinical Lectures: the Lectures of Carl Wernicke by Miller, R. and Dennison, J.)*. Heidelberg: Springer.

Weston, M. J., & Whitlock, F. A. (1971). The Capgras syndrome following head injury. *British Journal of Psychiatry*, 119, 25–31.

WHO. (1990). *Composite International Diagnostic Interview (CIDI) Version 1.0*. Geneva: World Health Organization.

Williams, E. B. (1964). Deductive reasoning in schizophrenia. *Journal of Abnormal Psychology*, 69, 47–61.

Wilson, M. (1993). DSM-III and the transformation of American psychiatry: a history. *American Journal of Psychiatry*, 150, 399–410.

Wilson, R. I., & Nicoll, R. A. (2001). Endogenous cannabinoids mediate retrograde signalling at hippocampal synapses. *Nature*, 410, 588–592.

Wilson, R. I., & Nicoll, R. A. (2002). Endocannabinoid signaling in the brain. *Science*, 296, 678–682.

Wing, J. K., Cooper, J. E., & Sartorius, N. (1974). *The Measurement and Classification of Psychiatric Symptoms*. Cambridge: Cambridge University Press.

Winokur, G. (1977). Delusional disorder (paranoia). *Comprehensive Psychiatry*, 18, 511–521.

Wise, R. A. (1978). Catecholamine theories of reward: a critical review. *Brain Research*, 152, 215–247.

Wong, D. F., Wagner, H. N., Jr., Tune, L. E. et al. (1986). Positron emission tomography reveals elevated D2 dopamine receptors in drug-naive schizophrenics. *Science*, 234, 1558–1563.

Woodward, T. S., Ruff, C. C., Thornton, A. E., Moritz, S., & Liddle, P. F. (2003). Methodological considerations regarding the association of Stroop and verbal fluency performance with the symptoms of schizophrenia. *Schizophrenia Research*, 61, 207–214.

Wustmann, T., Pillmann, F., Friedemann, J. et al. (2012). The clinical and sociodemographic profile of persistent delusional disorder. *Psychopathology*, 45, 200–202.

Yamamoto, K., & Hornykiewicz, O. (2004). Proposal for a noradrenaline hypothesis of schizophrenia. *Progress in Neuropsychopharmacology and Biological Psychiatry*, 28, 913–922.

Yin, H. H., & Knowlton, B. J. (2006). The role of the basal ganglia in habit formation. *Nature Reviews Neuroscience*, 7, 464–476.

Young, D., & Scoville, W. B. (1938). Paranoid psychosis in narcolepsy and the possible danger of benzedrine treatment. *Medical Clinics of North America*, 22, 637–646.

Zilboorg, G. (1941). Ambulatory schizophrenia. *Psychiatry*, 4, 149–155.

Zoli, M., & Agnati, L. F. (1996). Wiring and volume transmission in the central nervous system: the concept of closed and open synapses. *Progress in Neurobiology*, 49, 363–380.

Index

Printed in the United States
by Baker & Taylor Publisher Services